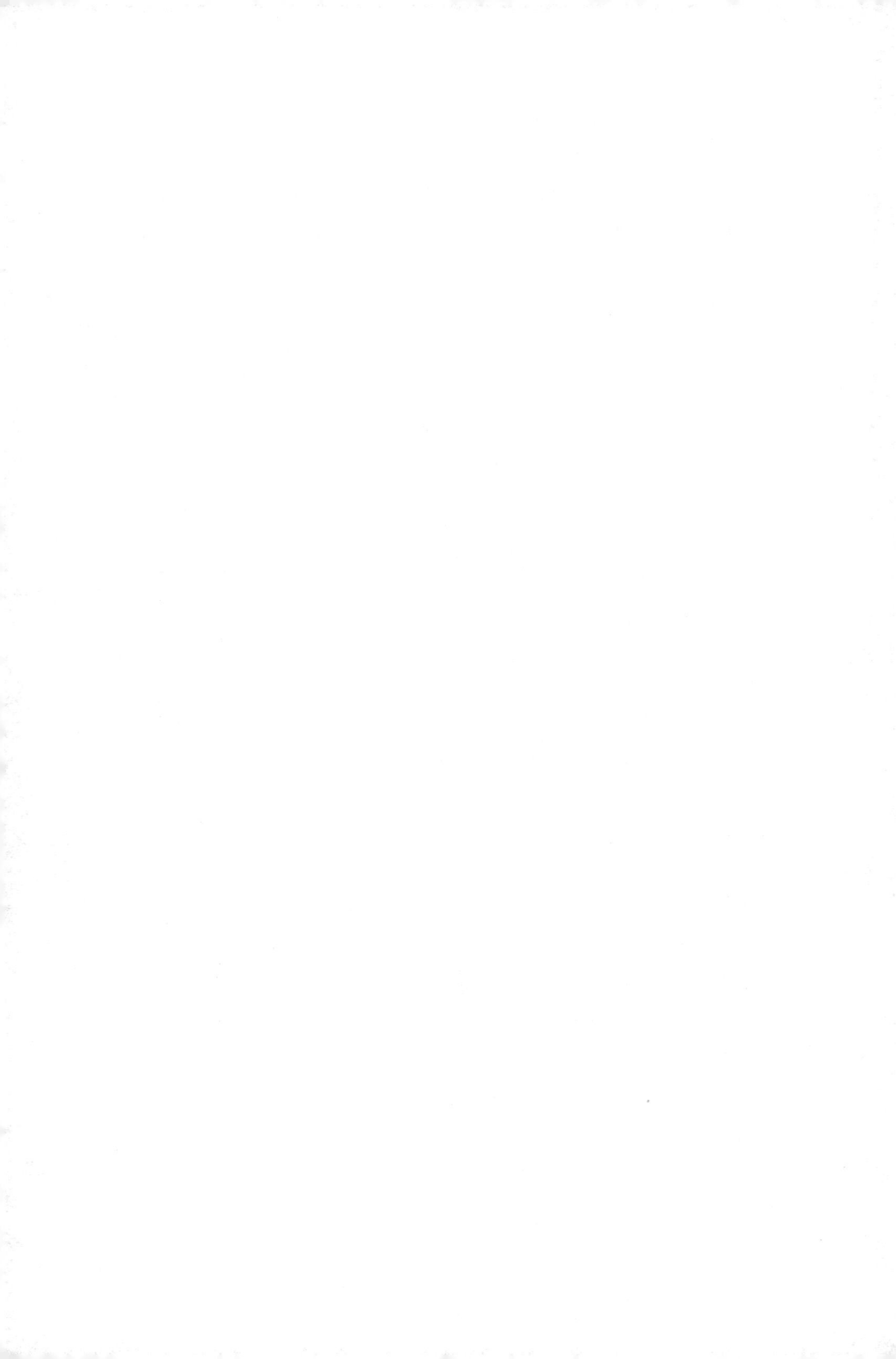

WHAT HEALTH ENTHUSIASTS ARE SAYING ABOUT OTILIA KISS...

"One day I met a beautiful woman who I believed was the happiest person I ever met. Very curious, I asked her for her secret to happiness. She only said: "What I eat makes me happy." In an instant, she gave me a green smoothie. I couldn't believe that bitter green thing could make anyone happy. Shortly after, I decided to make a change in my life and signed up for Otilia's 6-Month Personal & Health Development Program. I'm so happy and thankful for having chosen this path in my life. I learned, changed and accomplished so much! Now I take care of my physical body, my mind, and my emotions. Otilia gave me the tools to encourage myself to cultivate inner peace, self-esteem, and personal empowerment. And those tools really work! She helped me to change my body, my mind, my spirit, my mood, my energy, my digestion, my eating habits, my LIFE. I am so amazed at how my life has changed in the last six months. I feel like I am a completely different person. Thanks to her, my life 'tastes' different."

— *Liliana Becerril*

"I would like to thank Otilia for having shown me that there are no limits in life. I heard this so many times before, but she took my hand and literally walked me through the path of no limits. I am so grateful that she came into my life and changed it. I recently went to the doctor, and she said my B12 levels were now great and that I am a healthy person. The effect of our work still resonates!"

— *Blanca Cruz*

"As a client of Otilia Kiss for the past year and a half, I would not hesitate to recommend her as a nutritionist and life coach. Otilia is an incredible coach, mentor, nutritionist and all round soul. She is truly passionate about what she does and works hard and joyfully to help her clients reach their goals and evolve into their full potential. As a client, I felt cared about, supported, encouraged and inspired to keep moving forth. With her guidance, I have been able to achieve goals I had put my mind to and had an amazing coach to cheer me on all the way. I especially praise the fact that she takes a holistic approach, not only does she help clients with healthy eating and maintaining a healthy lifestyle but also helps clients to overcome limiting beliefs, helping us to feel and become empowered.

I would highly recommend investing in one of her Health & Life Coaching Programs, which has definitely been one of the best investments I have ever made and one of the best gifts I have ever given myself, the gift of true, vibrant health. Otilia truly goes above and beyond to help her clients achieve their goals. The program she offers is individually tailored, and throughout the challenges, Otilia made it an exciting, fun journey to be on."

—Valerie Le

"I have been diabetic for six years and taking medication to control it. My journey with Otilia began on my 56th birthday. By following her advice of what foods to eat and avoid, and following her schedule of nutrition and cleansing, I soon noticed my skin becoming brighter and having more energy. When the program ended, I conducted my second live blood cell test. The results astonished the technician. She had never witnessed someone having such extreme results. A secondary blood work revealed that I was almost free from diabetes.

Otilia helped me reduce my medications and feel healthy again, and I will never go back to the way I was eating in the past. I am truly grateful for what Otilia has done for me. I now have the health and energy to keep up with my grandchildren, and I know that I will be able to change them for years to come. Thank you!"

—Clara Noce

"I can't stress enough how powerful and informative Otilia's programs are! With the amount of overwhelming information out there that leaves me confused and frustrated, I have finally found concrete answers! Otilia's common sense and factual certainty in regards to health and food have finally made me see the truth with no doubts. After many years of blindly searching for the right guidance and information to be the healthiest we can be, we have finally found the right place."

—Renata Herceg

"My search for taking my vegetarian diet to the next level exceeded my expectations as I journeyed with Otilia and learned about making the best food choices. I always read labels before but this time with the awareness of choosing raw, organic and ingredients in their natural state. With this awareness, I was able to increase my iron levels and my intake of quality protein pre and post workouts. I also learned about new foods that enhanced my diet and helped me shed those extra pounds. This journey was also about me and reminding me about balancing everything that is important in my life. I am forever grateful to Otilia for her support and guidance."

—Cheryl D'Souza

From Trapped to Limitless

7 STEPS TO HEALTHY LIVING WITHOUT LIMITS

OTILIA KISS

Copyright © 2017 by Otilia Kiss

All rights reserved. No part of this book may be reproduced in any form or by any electronic or mechanical means, including information storage and retrieval systems, without permission in writing from the author. For information, contact Otilia Kiss at otilia@otiliakiss.com.

This book is not intended as a substitute for the medical advice of physicians. The reader should regularly consult a physician in matters relating to his/her health and particularly with respect to any symptoms that may require diagnosis or medical attention. Rather, it is intended to help you make informed decisions about your health and to cooperate with your healthcare provider in a joint quest for optimal wellness. Please consult your doctor for matters pertaining to your specific health and diet.

Although the author and publisher have made every effort to ensure that the information in this book was correct at press time, the author and publisher do not assume and hereby disclaim any liability to any party for any loss, damage, or disruption caused by errors or omissions, whether such errors or omissions result from negligence, accident, or any other cause.

Some names and identifying details have been changed to protect the privacy of individuals.

Mention of specific products, companies, organizations, or authorities in this book does not imply endorsement by the author or the publisher, nor does mention of specific companies, organizations, or authorities imply that they endorse this book. Internet addresses given in this book were accurate at the time it went to press.

To contact the author, visit:

WWW.OTILIAKISS.COM

Production Credits
Cover design: Pixelstudio
Interior design: www.bookclaw.com
Photographer: Gabi Starr
Printed by Create Space, An Amazon.com Company

ISBN-13: 978-1548686697

ISBN-10: 1548686697

This book is dedicated to all of you out there who have the same relentless hunger to learn, grow and be the best that you can be. May you never settle for anything less and may this book inspire you to create an even healthier and richer life for yourself and others.

CONTENTS

Foreword by Dr. Ashima Suneja-Chauhan, N.D. xv
Note To My Readers xix

STEP 1 WAKE UP! THIS IS THE ONLY LIFE YOU'VE GOT! 21
   Chapter 1.1 The Wake-Up Call 23
   Chapter 1.2 Awareness is Key - There Are No Limits Unless You Create Them 28
   Chapter 1.3 External Limitations 32
   Chapter 1.4 Internal Limitations 35
   Chapter 1.5 What's in Your Cake? Change Your Ingredients – Change Your Life 41

STEP 2 LET GO AND SEE THE POSSIBILITIES 47
   Chapter 2.1 Start Observing and Start Questioning 49
   Chapter 2.2 What Do You Really Want? 52
   Chapter 2.3 From Fear to Curiosity 57
   Chapter 2.4 Live From the End, As If You Already Have It 62

STEP 3 BUILD A STRONG FOUNDATION 65
   Chapter 3.1 Optimum Health Redefined 67
   Chapter 3.2 The Six Health Myths to Let Go Of 71

STEP 4 PLAY TO WIN – PICK THE STRATEGIES THAT WORK FOR YOU 83
   Chapter 4.1 Treat the Cause, Not the Symptoms. Your Lifestyle is Your Medicine! 85
   Chapter 4.2 Law #1: The Law of Optimum Hydration 90
   Chapter 4.3 Law #2: The Law of Maximum Nutrition 97
   Chapter 4.4 Law #3: The Law of Balanced Alkalinity 109
   Chapter 4.5 Law #4: The Law of Detoxification 113
   Chapter 4.6 Law #5: The Law of Movement 120
   Chapter 4.7 Law #6: The Law of Stress Management 125

STEP 5 PULL THE ANCHOR AND LEARN TO HANG ON ... 131
Chapter 5.1 Take Action Now ... 133
Chapter 5.2 Set Yourself Up for Success ... 137
Chapter 5.3 Sabotage is Inevitable ... 148

STEP 6 BUILD A SUSTAINABLE LIFESTYLE ... 157
Chapter 6.1 Don't Get Overwhelmed You Don't Have to Do It All ... 159
Chapter 6.2 You Will Find the "How" When You Are Ready ... 165
Chapter 6.3 Feed Your Mind ... 167
Chapter 6.4 Build Your Rituals Step-by-Step ... 170
Chapter 6.5 Always Have a Trick Up Your Sleeve ... 174
Chapter 6.6 Your Efforts Are Never Lost ... 179

STEP 7 LIVE IT! ENJOY IT! SHARE IT! ... 183
Chapter 7.1 Live Through Inspiration ... 185
Chapter 7.2 Listen When Your Soul Speaks ... 188
Chapter 7.3 The Journey to Your Dreams ... 190

The 7 Steps – Your Roadmap to the Health You Deserve ... 192
So Now What? ... 195
About the Author ... 197
Acknowledgements ... 199
Recommended Reading ... 201
References ... 203

From Trapped to Limitless

FOREWORD

Optimum Health. Wellness. Vitality.

These are all key concepts that have hit our health industry today – one of the leading industries in the world.

What is optimum health? What is wellness? What is vitality? The key is the absence of disease or discomfort in order to classify one as optimally healthy, well and vital. This permeates the mental, emotional and physical facets of life. If one is challenged mentally or emotionally, it creates dysfunction physically and vice versa. Our society has become one of convenience – we have moved so far from our natural rhythms – those same rhythms of the universe. We are simply microcosms of the macrocosm, and when our rhythms are out of sync, dysfunction arises. We are having such difficulty in adopting and maintaining healthy lifestyles because we want instant gratification – we do not want to work for ourselves. We have enslaved ourselves to working for big houses, expensive cars, popularity, riches – instead of prioritizing health and well-being at the top. Living the North American dream, coming to the land of opportunity, has robbed us of our health, well-being, and vitality. There's an old Indian proverb that says we work our entire lives to gain riches and when we have them, we spend it in trying to regain our health.

Growing up, I knew I wanted to be a doctor – to help those in need. I entered medical school and dropped out within the first year. I could not justify using pharmaceuticals as the only form of treatment. I knew in my heart that there had to be more to health than just drugs. I discovered naturopathic medicine purely by serendipity. After dropping out of medical school lost and searching, I found a little poster for naturopathic medicine tucked away in the corner of a career board. I hesitated, but went to an open house and immediately took to the idea. In my first year, I again had doubts and returned to visit my friends in medical school. In my week away from naturopathic medicine, I knew in my heart that I was intended to become a naturopathic doctor. And I haven't regretted a single moment of my pursuit. I have worked with hundreds of patients in my last decade of practice assisting and guiding them on their journey to optimum health, wellness and vitality. It is a true blessing and honor to be privy to these lives.

Otilia Kiss was one of these patients – she was working for a Fortune 500 company. Her stress levels were high, and her life was so busy that she would be running on empty all the time. Her adrenal glands were not functioning optimally, and she was losing steam. She continued to perform well at work, as this was her focus and her reason for staying in Canada. We were working on improving her diet, getting her sleep on schedule, managing her stress levels, and trying to keep up with her daily demands.

One day, she called me and told me that she quit her job and was enrolling in a Certification to become an Integrative Nutrition Health Coach. I knew that this was exactly what she needed to improve her life and most importantly to prioritize herself at the top of her list.

Fast-forwarding a few years, Otilia has become a speaker and entrepreneur and runs her own Health Coaching business teaching people how to live healthy and vibrant lifestyles. Otilia co-founded Thrive Organic Kitchen and Café, a health-focused restaurant with a vision to revolutionize the way people eat and to provide education and support for those looking to change their lives. Watching her in action at Thrive is enlivening – and confirms my thoughts that Otilia is on the journey to reach her optimum health, wellness, and vitality. Most importantly, Otilia has become one of the happiest people I know. A personal congratulations to you, Otilia.

As a means to pay it forward, Otilia has now written this book – From Trapped to Limitless. Interestingly, my name Ashima in the Hindi language means she who is limitless. So when Otilia asked me to write the forward of her book, I knew it was what I had to do.

This book helps individuals understand how to feel better, how to have more energy and how to enjoy life more. This book is geared to those who feel like they are not themselves like something is missing; they feel trapped and do not know how to move from that feeling. Individuals who aspire to do more with their lives and feel like their body cannot cope must read this book. This book provides hope and easy to implement solutions that can be integrated into life making optimal health, wellness and vitality possible and realistic. The mystery behind these ideas is unveiled to empower individuals with an understanding of the tools necessary to achieve long-term health, wellness, and vitality.

This book comes in a timely fashion when our society has swung so much in the direction of ill health and priorities furthest away from wellness. What's great about this book is that it allows the flexibility in choices and picking strategies that work for each individual, as opposed to laying out a cookbook one for all approach. Otilia walks the reader through seven steps to achieve optimum health and concludes with being limitless – living with awareness, through inspiration and imagining the unimaginable.

Personally, I have been through a similar journey – feeling trapped and unable to mobilize. There was an inner strength that allowed me to persevere, like Otilia, to reclaim my life with optimum health, wellness, and vitality – all without limits. I can see that this book can be a valuable tool to those wishing to live limitlessly. I wish Otilia and all her readers a life full of joy, happiness, optimum health, wellness, and vitality. And when challenges arise along the journey, finding the grace and flexibility to imagine the unimaginable.

— DR. ASHIMA SUNEJA-CHAUHAN, N.D.
Doctor of Naturopathic Medicine

NOTE TO MY READERS:

I have written this book to show you, my friends and readers, that you do not have to take for granted what you are being told, that the lifestyle you live, no matter what it may be, does not define you and does not limit the shape of your future health and well-being. You have a choice, and you can do something about it! The answer to any health-related challenge lies within you.

If you are ready to discover the real reason behind your pain or challenge, the first step is to stop looking outside of yourself, as the solutions are not there. All the money in the world, all the diet books, all the pills, all the healthy foods in the world and all the willpower in the world cannot help you get sustainable and long-lasting results. But you can! When you identify and break through all your inner and outer limitations, and you build a strong mindset and a strong foundation of health, you can make anything happen. Inspiring people to break through this invisible barrier is what I live for.

I strongly believe that the best healer in the world is you. You have everything you need to figure out what is good and what is not good for you. Stop being a patient. Stop listening to those who tell you that you cannot do it and stop taking everything you are being told for granted. Love yourself and value yourself every day. Take responsibility for your own life and live strongly and proudly knowing that you have done it all on your own.

My promise to you is that I will never try to fix you. Instead, I will do everything I can to empower you and support you so at any point in time you will know what to do without depending on anyone or anything. It's about putting the power and the choice back in your hands. It's not about diet shortcuts or the latest fad; rather, it is about learning to understand your body and your mind and get the tools and strategies that will help you make changes that can last forever.

This book is structured as a step-by-step journey, taking you from the moment a challenge is identified to the peace and tranquility that takes over your life when all is taken care of and healed. Let my own experience, and that of my clients guide you on this path. At the same time, visualize yourself in your journey and apply the techniques and strategies I share to get clarity on your unique health challenges.

I suggest that you first read the book in its entirety, then return to whichever step is most relevant to you and apply the strategies shared for as long as it takes to get the results you desire. There are no shortcuts, but there is always a way if you are truly committed. You don't always have to know how you'll get there; you just have to believe that you will.

Your health is the base upon which the rest of your life is built. I hope this book will inspire you and move you to discover and unleash the best version of yourself. It is waiting for you with love and anticipation for living the ultimate life. If you're with me, let the journey begin.

Otilia Kiss

STEP 1

WAKE UP!
THIS IS THE ONLY LIFE
YOU'VE GOT!

Chapter 1.1

THE WAKE-UP CALL

One moment can change a day, one day can change a life, and one life can change the world.

–BUDDHA

There was a moment in my life when I felt there was no hope and I simply saw no way out. I had spent the last thirty-one years living someone else's life, fighting for someone else's dream. And when I finally saw the truth, it felt like my whole life was falling apart in front of my eyes.

I had it all, but I had nothing because the one thing that truly mattered was threatened: my health, my well-being. The invisible energy that kept me moving for so long finally ran out one day when I awoke in the middle of the night in excruciating pain. It was the kind of pain you only hear about in books or someone else's story but never in your own. Most of my life I had lived in a self-created illusion where such unbelievable experiences could not possibly happen to me.

As I opened my eyes, I realized this was no dream. It was as real as it could possibly get. The pain on the left side of my abdomen was so strong that I could barely breathe. It felt like someone was stabbing me with a dozen knives. I felt completely out of control. As a friend was rushing me to the closest hospital, all I wanted to know was what could have happened to cause such an unexpected and painful experience. I had never been sick before. I had no symptoms, no sign of anything wrong happening inside my body.

Though I feared the worst, I was certain that the experts in the emergency room would have it all figured out in no time. An hour later, while still tossing in pain in the waiting room, my certainty slowly faded.

As though such experiences were normal, everyone around me seemed to follow the medical protocol to the letter: take a ticket, wait for your turn, register with the nurse, and come up with some sort of clear number from 1 to 10 to describe the pain experienced. At this point, I felt this question utterly surreal as I could barely hear any words or hold myself straight in the chair.

To my bewilderment, despite the fact that the number I picked was a 10, I ended up in a secondary waiting room, a few feet away from the first. I wondered what exactly would have to happen to get someone to see me. What followed next seemed to be an excerpt from one of my worst nightmares. After screaming in pain for over three hours, I was finally numbed up with a high dose of morphine. I have no recollection as to what happened next, as I passed out for the remainder of the night.

Even though that pain had truly been the worst in my life, what I experienced upon waking topped it off in a way I could not even fathom. I was told that I had an ovarian cyst that had burst and that such things were normal for women my age. I was to go home and take high-dosage sedatives for a few days to avoid the pain. There was nothing else necessary to be done, and I was reassured this was normal.

My mind was in overdrive mode trying to understand what this emergency room expert was telling me. Though I had no medical background myself, it just did not seem normal to me that this could happen to an apparently healthy person. I repeatedly asked for an explanation but to no avail. The answer was always the same. They did not know what caused it and I was to go home reassured that it was normal and that I would be okay. "We can't really do anything about it," the doctor said. "It's normal; it happens."

The sound of those words shook me to my core. I had heard them before, and here they were, coming back to haunt me again. I heard them in the words of my late grandmother who died of cancer and whose journey of disease began similarly with inexplicable cysts deemed to be normal by medical experts. I heard them before in the words of many family members who accepted their diseases as normal and as expected signs of old age. I heard them before in the words of our family doctor, who, for years and years, had been telling us that my severe anemia was nothing to be worried about.

Tears of anger started pouring down my face as the doctor handed me the drug prescription. And at that moment, something took over me, something that to this day I cannot explain. I looked at him...I looked at the sheet of paper...and I just said: "No! You cannot decide what my life will be! You cannot decide for me! I know this is not normal and I will figure it out!" This was my life, my only life, and no one and nothing was going to tell me how I was going to live it. "I can't just sit here and wait for the disease to show up," I thought.

I stood there in amazement at my own words, as I had no idea where they came from. I just knew that was not it. I knew there was more to this. I placed the drug prescription back into his hands and walked away. I stormed out that door with the most powerful feeling of determination I had ever experienced. I wasn't going to settle. I wasn't going to let anyone decide my life for me. I could have accepted someone else's words as my truth. I could have chosen to look at that experience as normal and do nothing about it. Instead, I saw it as an opportunity to grow and become more than I had ever been.

That fateful day was a major turning point in my life. It was a catalyst for change and for many magical moments that came my way in the years to follow. It opened my eyes to the reality that we are all facing, living our lives thinking that we have no control over our health, our thoughts, or our choices. This is why I am so passionate about inspiring you to break free of your fears and limitations, about showing you that there is another way. I cannot stand to see anyone limit their life, their health, their abilities, and their achievements because of the invisible barriers they don't realize they have or the self-created challenges they do not think they can overcome. I cannot stand to see someone not being able to live the life of their dreams because they are not aware of the limiting environment they unconsciously built around themselves. We were given this life to experience all that we can be, all that we can create, and all that we can share with those around us who wish to follow their dreams. We all have something unique to offer this world, and I truly believe that our mission in this life is to find it and share it with as many people as possible.

This powerful knowing is what drives me and feeds my mind, my body, and my soul every single day. It is the force that pushed me to write this book for those of you out there who have the same relentless hunger to learn, grow, and be the best that you can be. My dream is to inspire you to take action and radically transform your life and your health. I hope you'll let me be your guide and mentor on this wonderful journey. Together we'll break through the limitations and complexities of your current lifestyle and find the tools and resources that will help you build your dream life in an easy and sustainable way. You will come to know that when you take your health to the highest level possible, you can experience an abundance of energy beyond anything you can imagine right now. It is this powerful source of energy, this invisible life force that will allow you to do things you never thought possible. It is the base upon which the rest of your life is built. By the time you are done reading this book, you will have in your hands a clear step-by-step map to reclaiming your health and a set of principles that will support you in achieving and maintaining your health goals forever.

I know this may seem scary. I know this may seem crazy and impossible for you and your unique situation. But let me just say something from my heart to yours: to be successful in anything you want to do, you don't have to avoid the things that are too scary. You don't have to avoid the fear. You don't have to have a certain age or a certain degree or certification or an inborn talent. All you need is you! All you need is you making up your mind as to what you want and what makes you happy. You are not a victim of circumstances! You are the creator of your own life! Once you are clear on that, the rest is all a matter of learning to use your fears and limitations to push you forward instead of holding you back. It's all about finding the right tools and strategies that work for you.

You don't have to understand the science of nutrition to live a healthy lifestyle. All you need is an open mind and a sense of adventure. Today information is everywhere, and the truth is that we all know we need to eat better. And yet we don't. We allow ourselves to be caught in the net of countless to-do lists and responsibilities, putting our health aside and letting it drop to the bottom of our priority list. "We'll get to it some day" is too common a strategy in today's busy world.

So how do we begin to reverse all this?

The most powerful belief that guides my life is that there is always a way to get what you want if you truly want it, focus on it, and look for it. It is this strong conviction that ignited my desire to write this book and help you find that path for yourself. No matter how different our lives may be, there is a way for each one of us to achieve our goals (i.e. career goals, family goals, financial goals, etc.) while keeping our health a priority. It does not have to be one or the other. You do not have to choose. There is a way to have it all, and this book will show you how.

You have an opportunity here, my friends, at a brand new start. You have an opportunity to change the course you are on and continue on a better path. So don't wait until it is too late. Don't ignore the signs your body is sending you to let you know something is wrong. Let this be your wake-up call. Let this be that moment when you decide enough is enough; you can be more, and you will be more. If you are stressed and tired, you can find the tools to create more energy. If you feel depressed and overwhelmed you can learn new ways to feed your mind and change your perspective. If you feel like your mind and your body are stopping you from living your ideal life, you can learn new ways to reclaim your health once and for all. Everything is possible if you believe it so. All it takes is getting clear on what you want and deciding that you will not settle for anything less. There are no barriers unless you create them or unless you let others create them for you. It's time to say no to what doesn't serve you and to find out what you are truly capable of.

Chapter 1.2

AWARENESS IS KEY - THERE ARE NO LIMITS UNLESS YOU CREATE THEM

If you hear a voice within you say 'you cannot paint,' then by all means paint, and that voice will be silenced.

—VINCENT VAN GOGH

If you and I had met a few years back and you had told me of how I live my life today, what I learned, how I think, and most of all, how amazing I feel, I would have probably laughed in disagreement as back then I never thought anything like this was possible. I couldn't imagine being able to live and enjoy life this way. I couldn't imagine it because I had no references telling me otherwise. I thought that what I had experienced thus far was my reality and all that I was capable of. I had given my all in life, and that was as far as I could reach, I thought.

    So if you had met me back then, no matter what you had told me about how great I could feel, I wouldn't have believed you; I couldn't have believed you. How can you describe the smell of a rose to someone who has never smelt one? How do you tell someone how much clarity, energy, and vitality he or she can experience when their body is finally allowed and supported in working at its best? How do you even begin?

    If you find yourself feeling the same way as you read these pages, I would like to invite you to try something. First, don't fight back; let your feelings flow and observe. You do not have to agree with all that I say. All I will ask you to do is to notice and realize that you are reading this book because whatever you have done in the past to heal yourself has not worked. This book came your way because you are searching for a better way. Sometimes you cannot understand how life will turn out; sometimes you just have to take a leap of faith. Sometimes you have to pay attention to the signs and the people that are coming your way trying to point you in a different direction. The fact that you and I met or that you are reading my book is not a mere coincidence. It is one of life's beautiful arrangements to bring you onto your path and answer your call for help.

THE INVISIBLE BUBBLE

And so it all begins with you choosing to take a leap of faith into the unknown, into the possibility of a different way of living life. It all begins with you looking at your life and observing what is not working and what is holding you back from reaching your goals and dreams. Is it the way you feel emotionally? Is it the way your body feels? Is it your mind being tired or unfocused? Is it that you feel exhausted and can't seem to get yourself to do the things you love? Is it that your physical body just can't seem to keep up with all that you desire to do and achieve? Or is it that you know there is something more to life, but you just can't seem to get yourself to find out what it is?

Going through this process myself allowed me to understand that any time we find ourselves unable to move on past a certain point in our life, what is holding us back is not someone or something. It is a myriad of interlocked limitations, of negative beliefs, thoughts, emotions, and meanings from our inner and outer environment. This is what I call the invisible bubble of limitations that we are unaware of most of our lives. It is the continuous dance between our ability to see these limitations and our need to become more as human beings that will deeply affect our overall happiness and fulfillment and our ability to live the life we truly deserve.

What I came to realize, from my own experience and that of the people I had the privilege to work with during the last decade of my life, is that all these areas of our lives have one common thread. There is one area, in particular, that affects all others. It is the area of our health, our well-being. This is the one thing that can make or break anything else.

No matter how successful you may be in other categories of your life, I can promise you that, to some degree, not living in your optimum health zone is stopping you from reaching your greatest potential. You may want to take your business to the next level, but you feel you do not have the energy for it. You may want to work on your relationship, but you are too exhausted at the end of the day to give anything else to your partner. You want to be the best mom you can be, but you feel tired and overwhelmed and barely have enough energy to take care of yourself.

If you want more energy in your business – in other words, more progress, efficiency, and vitality – then you must first create it for yourself. If you want to be a better mom or partner, then you must take care of yourself first. The better you are, the better everything else will be. The more energy you have, the better you feel, and the better your business and your relationships will be. Living in your optimum health zone is the key to taking any other area of your life to the next level. It is the catalyst for change and the base upon which everything else in your life is built.

The first step to reaching your optimum health zone may be the most challenging, but it is lifting this anchor that gives you momentum, strength, and excitement to find new truths and set sail for a new direction in your life. To do so, you must first understand and become aware of the internal and external limitations and negative beliefs that are holding you back in this area of your life. You must first let go of the heavy baggage and break free. This takes looking back at your own life and finding the thoughts, ideas, and beliefs related to your health that you accepted as truths and allowed them to dictate every decision you made, every action you took or did not take and every result you got.

Breaking through these limitations and learning how to reach your optimum health zone does not have to be complicated. When you are clear on what you want, and you become aware of the universal laws that support optimum health, it all becomes easier, and you can learn to fall in love with every step of the process. At the end of the day, what really matters is not the destination but the journey itself. That's where the secret is. The day will come when you would have achieved everything on your list and what will truly matter at that moment is not the attainment of the goal itself but rather the person you grew to be in the process.

Let's begin by taking a closer look at what optimum health means for you right now and the sources from your inner and outer environment that shaped it into what it is today. Let's start peeling away the layers and identify some of the biggest barriers that have been stopping you or slowing you down from living as the best version of yourself.

Chapter 1.3

EXTERNAL LIMITATIONS

Your only limitation is the one you set up in your own mind.

−NAPOLEON HILL

We are all uniquely designed based on our biochemistry, our genes, our background, our blood type, our metabolic type, etc., and thus I believe that no one diet, one pill, nor one program can work for everyone. While it is true that we are what we eat, I also believe that we are what we drink, what we think, and the air that we breathe; we are the love in our life or the troubles in our life. Otherwise put, our health and well-being are deeply affected by the totality of the environment in which we live. Hence, looking at a holistic picture of your whole environment is essential to be able to start building your personalized road to health in an easy and sustainable way.

So what is your external environment comprised of?

It is the place where you live; it is your family, your relationships, your career, your thoughts, the TV channels you watch, the restaurants or grocery stores you have access to and the people you spend most of your time with. The notion that you are somehow limited in what you can achieve in the area of your health and physical well-being can come to you from many directions of your environment: overprotective parents who do not want you to fail the way they did, a stressful nine-to-five job that you do not love, a draining relationship that does not feed your heart and soul, a negative friend, your cluttered home, and even the limited food choices at your local grocery store.

How is it possible to reach your greatest potential in such a rigid and limiting environment? It is not; yet many people spend their whole life accepting this reality as it is, without questioning it. It's as if you live in a confining invisible bubble that limits the ways in which you can experience life.

To be able to see beyond and break free of this limiting bubble, you must first become aware of it. You must begin to question it and become open to the idea that what you can or cannot do is your own decision to make, not someone else's. You have a choice, and it is yours to make.

When we allow limiting external beliefs to enter our inner world, we can severely limit our view of what is possible to achieve. Instead of listening and paying attention to your outer world, pay attention to cues and messages from your inner self, your instinctual self. When you get clear on who you truly are, independent and unattached to anything or anyone around you, that's when you can truly start the journey to reclaiming your health.

Listen to your heart, not your head and not the people around you who, with the best of intentions, may cloud you with doubt due to their own fears and limitations. Just because it happened to them does not mean it will happen to you. No one and nothing can limit who you want to be unless you allow it.

Here are a few potential negative and limiting influences from your external environment to consider:
- Unsupportive friends or family
- Interacting with people who do not share the same goals and values as you
- Contradictory and complex information regarding nutritional needs
- Cluttered home or workspace
- Negative people at work or in social groups
- Stressful job
- Lack of access to healthy foods near work or home
- Negative events and situations
- Negative news overemphasized on the media
- Watching too much TV
- Microwaves
- Polluted environment

So ask yourself:

Who are you today because you have allowed things, events, situations, or people to limit your horizons, your actions, your whole being? Did you perhaps settle for a passionless relationship because you told yourself you couldn't do better? Did you maybe choose to work for a company instead of building your own enterprise because your parents told you that was the more secure way to earn an income? Did you perhaps put your health aside because life got too busy and you simply couldn't find the time? Or did you maybe choose a lifeless, toxic meal for lunch simply because there were no other choices?

Whatever it may be, know that you are the one sitting in the driver's seat of your own life and that gives you one unique advantage. You and only you can choose at any time to pull the brakes and change your course. While it may be challenging to push the brakes after years of allowing fears and limitations to run your life, once you stay on the path for a while you will gain momentum, and your progress will only get easier.

Chapter 1.4

INTERNAL LIMITATIONS

Believe in yourself and all that you are. Know that there is something inside you greater than any obstacle.

—CHRISTIAN LARSON

You want to start exercising, but you find too many excuses not to begin. You tell yourself you want to change, but it seems too overwhelming, so you never actually follow through. You want to eat better but you think you will feel deprived of your favorite foods and that would be too painful. You want to lose weight, but you feel you don't know how. Nothing seems to work.

Does any of this sound like something you ever experienced?

Here's the first great news: it is not your fault; it's something else that you may not even be aware of. The root cause of your failure to take action on your desires is a bouquet of beliefs about what you can and cannot do. The beliefs we hold in any area of our lives are a result of our childhood programming. As children, we come into this world with an empty canvas that quickly gets filled up with information from anyone and anything in our environment. It is this programming that dictates what we think, what we believe, and the actions we take or don't take.

If you truly want to change the current state of your health, then you must divorce all negative beliefs you currently have about health. It is those beliefs that have brought you to exactly where you are today. Thinking that this is reality, that this is just the way things are, that there is nothing you can do about it, is a limiting belief that will not allow you to transcend your current state and take charge of your health. You must change it with one that will empower you to move on.

So if you currently feel like you are not making progress, like you are stuck and cannot see the way out, it's because of a story made up of thousands of beliefs that stop you from taking action and making progress. Let's say you believe that the reason you do not exercise is that you do not have time for it. Is that true? You may say that it's not, but in fact, it is true if you believe it so. It is true for you! Whatever you believe, whether it is true or not, whether it serves you or not, it becomes your truth, your reality. It is the root cause of any decision you make or don't make.

The second piece of good news is that you can change your beliefs should you wish to do so. You can decide right here and right now that you are more than what you did or were in the past. You are more than what others told you that you could be. Your abilities are not based on past performance or the limitations of your inner and outer environments, as we discussed in the previous chapter. Instead, they are based on your present focus and decisions.

One of the things I heard over and over again in my childhood was that I was too nice and too kind to have a career in business, as people would take advantage of me and not take me seriously. Somehow my family had related, in their minds, the concept of one being kind and nice to having these qualities hinder one's ability to be successful in this field. Instead, I chose to believe that my ability to be kind and positive was a key strength that would give me the unique advantage of seeing the world around me with different eyes. And so it did. Had I chosen to accept my family's limiting beliefs, perhaps I would have never been able to complete a business degree, become my previous employer's youngest district manager in the country, and, today, a successful entrepreneur and business owner.

Your beliefs about what may or may not happen, may cloud your ability to identify the facts in any given situation. Some beliefs are severely limiting in that they do not allow you to get a clear interpretation of a situation, person, or act. We often filter those experiences through our own lens that is made up of limiting thoughts and emotions. The good news is that you can change your lens, you can change the filters through which you evaluate your own abilities. And you certainly are not stuck living the rest of your life within the confines of your current reality.

Whatever state of health you are currently in, it is because of the totality of beliefs that you have about it. But don't just take what I say for granted. Try it! Let's say, as an example that you want to lose some weight and get fit but have not been able to reach your goal. Take a look at the questions below and mark down the ones you answered with a "yes."

- Do you believe you are not good enough to figure out this issue?
- Do you believe the nutrition industry is too complex and you do not understand it?
- Do you believe you may fail again because you did in the past?
- Do you believe you don't have the necessary genes?
- Do you believe it will be too painful?
- Do you believe you don't deserve to look and feel great?
- Do you believe it won't last, so why bother?
- Do you believe you don't have time for it?
- Do you believe you need money to make it happen (e.g. to hire a trainer or join a gym) and you don't have that kind of money right now?
- Do you feel like the gym is too far?
- Do you feel like the whole thing of going to the gym seems too overwhelming? (i.e. you have to remember to pack your things every time, drive all the way there, change your clothes, spend an hour sweating like a dog, shower, get dressed again, fix your hair, and then head on the long drive home?)
- Do you believe fit and healthy people are just "lucky" and you are not?

If most of your answers were yesses, then it is clear where the problem is. It's not time, it's not money, it's not the lack of proper clothing, it's not distance, nor is it your ability; it's your beliefs. So take a deep breath and just think about that for a second. It's not you; it's your beliefs where the true challenge lies. The great news is that you can change those the moment you decide to do so. You can take control of your actions and results from the moment you change your beliefs about them.

What if you did not believe any of the above and instead you believed that you were worthy, able, and truly committed and that nothing could stand in your way to achieving your health goals? Not time, not money, not distance, not anything. Would you do it then? I bet you would! Because then it would become a must and you would make it a priority above all else.

Here is a list of some of the most powerful positive beliefs that I used to help my clients and myself in building a new path towards optimum health.

- My health is the base upon which my life is built.
- I am larger than any health challenge I could ever face.
- Nothing tastes as good as healthy feels.
- Nothing tastes as good as being fit feels.
- What I knew about being healthy is not necessarily true. I choose to adopt new ways of thinking that support me on my journey to optimum health.
- I release any disempowering beliefs about my health from the past, and I create a new future filled with energy, vitality, and strength.
- I am committed to eating the healthiest food possible, as nothing is more important to me than my health.
- I have and deserve the very best in my life right now.
- I love myself completely and take excellent care of my mind and body.
- I let go of all that I no longer need. My body is healing quickly and easily.
- I rest peacefully every night knowing that my body knows what to do to heal while I sleep.
- My source of energy is abundant and never-ending.

A printable list of these empowering beliefs is available for download at www.otiliakiss.com in the Free Resources section. Print the sheet and place it everywhere you can see it: in your washroom, shower, and kitchen, on the door of your house, in the car, in your office, on your computer desktop or as reminder on your phone. Read the statements or say them out loud every day, morning and night. Make them a part of your life. Do whatever it takes to live and breathe these new thoughts as much as you can for as long as you can. Before you know it, you will find yourself making new decisions, trying new things, and taking actions in new and exciting ways. I've done it, my clients have done it, and so can you.

One of my clients, Amelia, had been diagnosed with Type 2 Diabetes a few years before we met. Though she drastically changed her food intake while we were working together, she was in desperate need of exercising to wake her body up and activate her internal healing system. She had never done much exercise in her life and was intimidated by the belief that she would have to work out for hours weekly in order to achieve the results she desired. It felt too overwhelming for her and, as expected, she never followed through. The simple strategy that changed everything was the idea that she could work out at whatever level she was at. This is what it means: If you are a beginner, you cannot work out in a healthy way by doing what a seasoned person would do. You can start as small as you need to. If all you can do is five minutes a day, then that's all you have to do.

Changing her beliefs about this was extremely liberating for her and allowed her to achieve great results quickly. She went from doing nothing to incorporating simple exercises around her house every day. The more she did, the better she felt and the more she was able to push herself. Before you know it, she was attending weekly yoga and Zumba classes and was able to reduce all her diabetes markers drastically.

Had she chosen to stick to her old beliefs, she would have never been able to bring such a positive change in her lifestyle. Her transformation was remarkable. At the halfway mark in our program, while revisiting her initial goals, she found she had already surpassed anything she ever thought possible – all because she chose to believe in something better, something that gave her a chance to reverse years of damage.

Choose to believe in yourself. Choose to love yourself and choose to accept the truth that you can change all that does not serve you. Don't limit yourself to what your family or friends or school or your culture tell you that you can or cannot do. Though motivated by the purest of intentions, they may not understand you, your strengths, and what you are truly capable of. Don't limit yourself by believing that's all there is. There is always more no matter what anyone tells you. We tend to believe in experts, but we never question what makes someone an expert. Is it a degree, a certification, a paper that says you went to school for four years?

Don't pay attention to negative patterns of thought that come as a result of what we have been conditioned into believing. Start questioning all of that and start listening to signals sent from your inner self and your instinctual self. It will tell you what to do because you and only you know what you need and what is best for you. Let's stop taking for granted what we are given and stop being ignorant to the desperate signals our body is sending us in its attempt to heal itself.

I believe expertise is ingrained in all of us, whether we have a paper proving so or not. If we learn to listen carefully, our bodies tell us what they need all the time. It can be as simple as knowing that feeling tired means you need to rest more, to something more complex such as pains, aches, and symptoms that all together point to a deeper source that you need to heal. Our body speaks to us all the time, but we can't hear it when we live in a bubble of limiting thoughts and beliefs. We have been taught all along to listen to others instead of listening to what comes from within, from our true self. We need to begin to let go and to switch our attention from our outer self to our inner self. That's when true magic begins to happen.

Chapter 1.5

WHAT'S IN YOUR CAKE? CHANGE YOUR INGREDIENTS – CHANGE YOUR LIFE

Everybody is a genius. But if you judge a fish by its ability to climb a tree, it will live its whole life believing that it is stupid.

—ALBERT EINSTEIN

As a little girl, I grew up in a family of doctors and pharmacists. I remember often being told how lucky I was because of that but I never quite understood why. Everywhere I looked there was someone sick. Many of the people in my life suffered from heart disease, debilitating constipation, liver damage, anemia, exhaustion and several other symptoms that are far too many to enumerate. My family seemed to own an entire drugstore as pills of different shapes and colors filled the house.

We never left anywhere without the "pill bag." I remember times heading out to town or on a trip and the bag was always there. "Just in case," they would say. There seemed to be almost an invisible dependency on this bag of what they called "the helpers." Every single symptom had its assigned pill. No matter what came up, there was something designed for it. It was almost as if disease and illness were expected and that they were sure to arrive at some point in time.

And so, for a long time, getting healthy for me was nothing more but the precise alignment of multicolored 'pellets' to whatever 'abnormal behavior' our body would every so often exhibit. As a child, health for me was not about the absence or prevention of disease. Rather, it was about waiting for it and being ready upon its arrival. I recall being sick more often than not, hit by throat infections, severe fever, and nausea. By seven years of age, my legs had deep scars from the hundreds of injections that I had received, and my gut had been destroyed due to the never-ending array of antibiotics.

As years passed by and my understanding of the human body expanded I began noticing some patterns that simply did not make sense to me. If the "magic pill bag" was there to address our body acting up, then why was it that it acted up to begin with? No matter whom I turned to, they always seemed to have an elusive answer. "It's just the way it is," they would say.

As a teenager, I remember rebelling against taking medicine more than I ever protested for not being allowed to go out or have a boyfriend. By this point, I was on a mission to refuse any pill. Though I had no idea what caused disease, all the little signs I had seen so far were clearly pointing out that bags of magic pills were not the solution. "What if there was no disease to begin with?" I would ask. "What if our bodies never acted up? Where does illness come from?"

My never-ending quest to find out the hidden source of disease set me on a course that would change my life forever. Though I had no idea at the time, those early childhood moments wondering and questioning this source triggered a new course and shape in my life. Today I cannot possibly be more grateful for the lessons that shaped who I am.

In a strange and inexplicable way, the horrific pain I experienced when my ovarian cyst burst needed to happen so as to push me to change, to push me to look for answers and never to take for granted my mind and my body. At thirty-one years of age, in that hospital room, I was once again listening to those words that were so painfully sprinkled all throughout the early years of my life. "You can't, we can't, I can't..." were so deeply embedded in my psyche that the mere sound would cause chills up my back and tears in my eyes. "Who are you to tell me what to do?" my soul would ask. "Who are you to set such invisible limits to what I wish and desire to do?"

These questions were implanted in the deepest corners of my mind and never left me to this day. They helped and supported me to break through barriers I could have never imagined. They revealed to me a new world of limitless possibilities as well as invisible barriers that our external and internal environment often sets for us.

Today I no longer prepare myself by filling my bag with magic pills; instead, I uplift my mind, my body, and my soul with tools and strategies that allow me to grow stronger every day. I don't wait for disease to show up. Instead, I focus on building a base upon which my life can stand strong no matter what comes my way. This is what you are also capable of doing, and it all starts with looking back at your own programming to figure out the exact thoughts and beliefs that are limiting you from living as your higher self.

Take a moment now and think about your childhood programming and how it affected your own choices and path in this area of your life.

- What did you learn about health when you were little?
- What did you observe concerning your close family or friends?
- What did you learn in school?
- Was there anyone in your family who had a health challenge similar to yours?
- What did you learn from that person about that particular issue?

Take a few minutes and dig deep to get some clarity, as this will reveal the hidden source of every thought, action, or decision you ever took in the area of your health. Capture your thoughts in a journal and continue to update the list as you make progress in the chapters to come.

A couple of years ago I completed this exercise with one of my clients, Christina. She reached out to me, desperately looking for help to lose weight. She felt like she had tried every diet plan she could get her hands on, but nothing worked. She would lose the weight for a while and then it would slowly creep back on even more than before. During our work together she discovered some extremely limiting beliefs about her ability to lose weight that she learned when she was just a few years of age. One of her close family members had had a weight challenge all her life and always used to say that it was in her genes and there was nothing she could do about it. Christina did not realize that subconsciously she never truly believed that she could lose the weight, and so she set herself up for failure without realizing. Once she identified this limiting belief, she was quickly able to let it go and learn that, despite our genes, many people can find ways to live a healthy life in a way that works for their unique body and biochemistry. She found the tools and strategies that worked for her and built an empowering environment that allowed her to achieve the weight she desired and maintain it indefinitely.

The principles for losing weight and keeping it off in the long term are the same as dealing with any other chronic illness. Before you can figure out how you to resolve it, you must trace it back to its original roots to understand what created it and what negative programming has allowed it to exist for so long. Shedding light on the roots of your challenge and the limiting beliefs around it will begin to slowly break down the power of any excuse or limitation that has been keeping you away from solving it.

Deep awareness of your health challenge will take away some of its grip on you and open up the door to new possibilities for getting it resolved. In the following chapter, we will begin to look at what is possible for you and help you see new options and ways to address whatever health challenge you may have. The answers are there for you to see the moment you change the lens through which you look at the world.

STEP 1 – Key Takeaways

1. Know that the best health expert in the world is you, and no one else can truly know what is best for you. Learn to listen to your body, your mind, and your soul and all the answers you are searching for will be revealed to you.
2. Stop looking for shortcuts and start focusing on enjoying the journey towards reaching any goal that you may have. The secret to fulfillment lies in your journey.
3. Never take your health for granted. Your body is your temple and the vehicle that you were given for expressing yourself in this life. The better your body and your health (i.e. physical, mental, emotional, spiritual), the better you will be, and the more amazing this life experience will become.
4. Start paying attention to people, situations, words, thoughts, beliefs, and feelings that hold you back from going after the things you want.
5. Start paying attention to health-related limitations such as feeling tired, depressed, unfocused, or lacking energy and drive. Never accept these as "normal" and avoid anyone telling you that it is okay to feel that way because of your age, gender, culture, genetics, etc.
6. Your beliefs shape who you are; they are at the core of any decision you make or don't make.
7. You are in control of your beliefs the moment you choose so. You can change them anytime you want in a way that empowers you to follow your dreams.
8. Start paying attention to what beliefs you hold in the area of health and how they make you feel. If I say to you right now to put on a pair of running shoes and go out for a jog, what kind of emotions do you instantly feel? What are the beliefs that come up? Feel them, see them, and know that you can change them anytime you wish to do so.
9. Here is a simple "Limiting Beliefs" exercise to help you achieve just that.

a. Take a few minutes and make a list of all negative beliefs you have in the area of health.
b. Write them on the left side of a sheet of paper.
c. Then ask yourself: what would you need to believe in order to do the necessary things for achieving your health goals? What new belief would you need to acquire?
d. Write these new positive beliefs on the right side of the paper even if you feel like you do not believe them at this moment.
e. Keep this new list with you anywhere you go. Read the new empowering beliefs at least three times daily. In a short time, you will see amazing things happen as new and positive beliefs begin to settle in.
10. We are all different, and no one thing can work for everyone. One's source of healing can be another's source of pain. Your personal level of optimum health is what you need to strive for.

Recommended Reading: *The Magic of Believing* by Claude M. Bristol

STEP 2

LET GO AND SEE THE POSSIBILITIES

Chapter 2.1

START OBSERVING AND START QUESTIONING

Question reality, especially if it contradicts the evidence of your hopes and dreams.

—ROBERT BRAULT

A few years ago I was in a rut. I had just entered into the fifth year of a dead relationship. I was working 12-hour days in the basement of an old building with no fresh air or natural light. Like many people these days, I was stressed, tired, depressed and simply saw no way out.

Do you ever feel like you are sliding down a wormhole covered in slime and no matter what you do, you cannot find anything to hold on to? The deeper you go, the more impossible it seems to get out. Well, I did feel this way for a long time – so long, in fact, that at some point I almost gave up.

Like many things in life, sometimes we have to hit rock bottom before we can push ourselves up. Otherwise, it's just not painful enough. The challenge for me was that I never quite hit rock bottom. I always seemed to linger somewhere in between, like a hoverboard on water, not high enough to take flight and low enough to sink. And, sadly, this is the most dangerous place to be. It is a comfort zone that is extremely difficult to escape.

One day I was sitting exhausted on my couch after a long day at work and, as always, tossing around in my head the same negative thoughts I had been focusing on for the last few years, all with the same result: anxiety, stress, sadness, etc. I remember telling myself that I had tried it all, that there was nothing else that I could do. None of the strategies I could think of to escape my situation seemed to give me any promising prospects.

In sheer desperation over my inability to think my way out of that mess, I left my house and went for a long walk. It was a windy fall day, and the drying leaves of the beautiful Canadian maple trees seemed helpless against the force of the wind. No matter how hard they tried, the leaves would fall, and a new cycle would begin. If they were going to be aligned with the course of nature, they had no choice but to let go and let be; they had no choice but to stop interfering with the natural ways of nature.

As I was watching this beautiful transformation of nature unfold, I got the answer I was so desperately looking for. It had been there in front of my eyes all this time. I had to let go. I had to stop interfering and allow nature to take its course. I was trying to force it to go in a direction that it was not ready to go in, a direction that maybe did not have my best interests in mind. All I had to do was trust and allow myself to be. I had to change from forcing to allowing, from "doing" to just "being." That moment was a crucial stepping stone in my life as, for the very first time, it allowed me to get out of the bubble I had built around myself and explore a new world of possibilities.

The most useful aspect of this process is the idea of not interfering with the course of nature, the course of life. If you ever catch yourself being so out of control, remember that the most important thing you can do is not to fight it; just go with it and watch, observe, and be aware of where it is taking you. Without interference, you will be able to remain impartial and make decisions out of anticipation, not reaction.

Trying to control people, events, and circumstances puts you in a limited reality bubble that is hard to escape. This rigid and stressful bubble is filled with negative beliefs, experiences, events, and feelings from the past. The more we focus on them, and the more we analyze them, the more there are. Thoughts like "I am not good enough" or "I am not worthy enough or confident enough or smart enough or old enough" fill our bubble like a seemingly unstoppable stream of water that we feel helpless against. They come from everywhere, from our parents who in an attempt to protect us from harm pass on their own fears to us, from an educational system based on rewarding some children but not all, or from health experts trained to subdue our symptoms instead of helping us get rid of the source of the problem.

The only way out is to stop fighting; let the sand settle and begin to observe. Just breathe calmly and look around. Listen to your inner voice, your inner wisdom, that part of you that keeps you breathing and staying alive. And begin to question everything you see. Ask yourself: "What is happening in my life right now that simply does not make sense?"

- Does it make sense that I spend more than 50% of my day in a cluttered office with no fresh air?
- Does it make sense that I cannot control my cravings for fried or processed foods?
- Does it make sense that I drive two hours a day in crazy and polluted traffic?
- Does it make sense that I cannot remember the last time I did something I loved?
- Does it make sense that I spend my life in a relationship that I know with utmost certainty is doomed?
- Does it make sense that I spend more time at work than with my loved ones?
- Does it make sense that I cannot spare an hour a day to work out and take care of my body?

You know deep in your heart that none of these make sense. And even though you may not have an idea right now as to how you could escape such a reality, just know that by the simple fact of noticing your bubble, you are far ahead of so many who never bother looking. You are light years ahead of many who take it all for granted and never question what they are being told or what they experience.

Chapter 2.2

WHAT DO YOU REALLY WANT?

Clarity is power. The more clear you are about what you want, the more likely you are to achieve it.

—BILLY COX

Whenever I start working with new clients, I always ask them to describe their health goals to me. Some say they want to lose weight; some want to have more energy, some want to detox and so on. Those answers are good but I know there is always something more to it and so I dig a little deeper. I ask them: "Okay, how much weight do you want to lose?" or "What do you wish you were able to do with more energy that you cannot do now?" or "Why do you feel you need to complete a detox program?"

Most often than not, I get no clear answer. The truth is that many of us don't have a clearly defined idea of what we want. Our goals are often vague or not specific enough. What are the chances that you will ever get something if you don't really know what it is, how it is and why you want it? Your chances are pretty much slim to none. Not impossible, but definitely not guaranteed.

CLARITY IS POWER

Not too long ago we celebrated the holiday season, and I was helping my stepdaughter Athena to write her letter to Santa. Of all things, she wanted a "real" gecko. Geez, I thought, I'd better make this as clear as possible; otherwise, Santa might not know exactly what she meant by that. I seriously did not want a live creepy-crawly to show up under our tree if you know what I mean...So I asked her to describe her desired gecko in as much detail as possible. And let me just say, she had absolutely no problem doing so. It was like this and like that, and it had to have this and that, and it had to be able to move his feet a certain way and wiggle his tail in another way etc....Wow! I did not even have a clue before that toy geckos could do all those things or that they even existed. But they did! They did, in her imagination!

So why is it that as adults we don't seem to be able to describe our goals in such a specific and measurable way? Is it because we just assume they will happen anyway? Is it because we don't really believe that they will come true, so we don't even bother? Whatever the reason is, reality shows that we need to do a better job at it if we are to get the things we say we desire, whether it's losing weight, feeling better, learning how to switch to a vegan lifestyle or just getting more fit. We have to make our goals specific, attainable, and measurable. Here is an example of two possible ways to describe your goal of losing weight:

NOT TO DO
I want to lose weight.

TO DO
I want to lose 10 pounds in 4 months.
I want to fit in my size six jeans.

If you were to accomplish this goal, would you know that you did? Yes, you would! It is because you made it very specific and measurable. It's not a vague amount of weight in a vague amount of time; it is 10 pounds in 4 months. It is also realistic as 10 pounds in that time frame is safe and truly achievable. It is also measurable as you can check the scale and use the size six jeans to know.

Does this make sense? I hope it does, as this is a crucial step for you to understand so that moving forward there are no gray areas when it comes to what it is you want in life. It is these kinds of gray areas that help shape the limiting bubbles we discussed in the previous chapter. Not knowing what we want with clarity stops us or slows us down from achieving it. And sometimes we can even reach our goal without realizing that we did.

REASONS HAVE POWER

Years ago, before I had embarked on my new and healthy lifestyle, I was on a different path and a different journey. I wanted to be healthy, fit, and vibrant, just like I do now, but there was something significantly different. Though I knew what I wanted and I was very clear and specific about it, I was never able to achieve my goals the way I wanted. I would reach my desired weight or energy for a while, but it would not last. It always felt like I had to struggle to stay there. I was stuck, hovering slowly between being too skinny or too fat to being too overwhelmed or too tired to do anything about it.

I remember one day I was complaining to one of my friends about my inability to maintain consistent results and she asked me with curiosity: "Why do you want this so badly?" It is rare for me to be rendered speechless. In this case, I was, and I didn't really know why.

The more I thought about it, the more I realized that the reasons I wanted to be healthy and fit had nothing to do with me and my personal vision of my life. I was doing it because someone said I should or because of social expectations and perhaps a limiting belief that who I was as a person was directly linked with how my body looked. Once I got clear on this, it became very obvious to me why I had not been able to achieve consistent results. Not only was I not clear on why I was doing it but also my "why" was linked to someone else's beliefs and not my own. This made all my reasons weak and therefore not able to get me from where I was to where I wanted to be.

If you've gotten this far in my book, it is clear to me that you have a very strong desire to take charge of your health and you want to be the best that you can be. But do you know *why*?

Take a moment and think about this. Review the following questions and potential answers and see which ones, if any, you identify with:

- Why do you want to take charge of your health?
- Why do you want to lose weight or get over an illness or have more energy?

Potential answers:
- o Because my doctor told me that I had to.
- o Because my partner told me that he or she wished I was more fit.
- o Because I feel I have to keep up with my peer group, where everyone is fit and healthy, and I don't want to be different.
- o Because everyone says I have to be skinny to be successful.
- o Because I cannot love myself until I am fit and healthy.

As you may realize already, these are limiting and negative beliefs that do not have the power to get you long-lasting results. In this case, your *why* is connected to something outside of you. External pressure may work for a while, but sooner or later you will find yourself going back to your old habits.

Take a look at the questions and possible answers below and see if you can feel the difference.

- Why do you want to take charge of your health?
- Why do you want to lose weight or get over an illness or have more energy?

Potential answers:
- o Because I truly believe that the healthier and stronger I am, the more I have to give to all those I love.
- o Because I know deep in my heart that this is the only life I've got and I want to live it the best way possible.
- o Because I want to be a role model for my kids, my family, and my friends as to what is truly possible when one is committed to living as their higher self.

Can you see how, in this latter example, your *why* is connected to something within you? It is linked to you becoming more as a person. In this case, it will be strong enough to give you lasting results. The better you are, the more you have to share with others. It will allow you to have better relationships, to have more fun with your children, to perform better at work, and to have energy left at the end of the day to do the things you love, not just the things you feel you have to do.

Having a powerful, positive, and supportive *why* that comes from within is essential for you to achieve any goal in life, be that in the area of health or any other aspect. I know that, if you are reading these words right now, it is because you are not happy with something and you are looking for solutions to resolve it. I truly honor you for that, and I promise you that you are light years ahead of those who never look or those who give up too soon.

Take some time right now to go back to the moment when you decided to purchase this book. You wanted to improve something about your health. Whatever your goals are, think about your reasons for wanting to achieve them. Why do you want to lose weight or get over a chronic problem? What will you gain if you decide to take massive action towards its attainment? How will your life change for the better? Before you move on to the next chapter, take a moment and jot down your answers. Reviewing these on a daily basis will help you build a strong sense of certainty and belief that everything you wish to achieve is possible. Positive, empowering beliefs are your key to success!

Chapter 2.3

FROM FEAR TO CURIOSITY

Who seeks shall find.

−SOPHOCLES

Six years ago I had finally reached a point where I was ready to take my health and well-being to the next level. I was ready to escape my makeshift bubble and move on. But no matter how much I tried, something seemed to hold me back. I was looking for the door, looking for a way out, and could not find it.

What was clouding my view at the time is the same reason for which many of us never seem to be able to take that very first step into a new experience. It was the fear of the unknown, and it was the belief that I did not know how to do so. These two powerful forces were tied around me like a rope with no end and no beginning.

I was afraid I would fail; I was afraid I would once again prove that I was not good enough and that all of those who did not believe in me were right. And if somehow I managed to pull through this fear, I would hit another wall, that of the debilitating feeling of not knowing how to do something.

How would I break free?
How could I leave this relationship?
How would I survive?
How would I drop all the foods I was addicted to?
How would I get myself to work out every day when I hadn't done so ever in my life?

No matter how much I asked and no matter how much I pushed myself to come up with an answer, I only seemed to be resisting it even more. And so I said to myself: "Well, I've got nothing to lose; I made it to the point where I can see my bubble so there must be something that I did right." And so I decided to apply the same principle as before and focused on not resisting. The more I let go, the less pressure I felt. I just went with the flow, watching and observing my world with a renewed sense of curiosity.

I began observing all the things that I was so afraid of and got curious about them. I did not force myself to change. Rather, I told myself to just go with it. I kept looking for things that did not make sense, for events, people, and situations that I was not used to seeing. And the more I looked, the more I saw.

Every day something new appeared: a strange-looking green drink at my usual café, a random Facebook post about a new personal empowerment group in my area, a new training course at work that focused on emotional intelligence, and new people who seemed to be altogether positive and truly fulfilled. Though I did not completely understand the meaning of all this, I never stopped watching, analyzing, and staying curious about them. Every once in a while I would peek through even deeper and try a new drink, read the health pages of a random wellness magazine, or engage in a conversation with someone who knew a thing or two about this mysterious world of nutrition.

It all seemed like a world I did not understand, but something inside me told me to keep going and never look back. And so I did. Today, after having spent years studying wellness, life coaching, and other health improvement techniques, I can clearly see that somehow, though I had no idea what I was doing at the time, I instinctively applied one essential principle that helped me take quantum leaps towards achieving my health dreams and goals. The principle was this: Dance with your fears!

If you are afraid of something, do not force fear; don't lie to yourself by saying that you are not afraid. Thank your mind for activating these feelings in you, as all it is trying to do is protect you from harm, not knowing the difference between a dangerous or harmless situation. Allow fear to be as it is and move together with it into a state of curiosity and intrigue. Ask a lot of questions about anything that does not make sense to you or anything that is new and interesting.

The more curious you get about your health related fears, the more new possibilities will start heading your way.

THE MYSTERIOUS BAGEL

One day, a co-worker of mine showed up at work with something fascinating in her lunch bag. It was a kind of bagel I had never seen before. It was not quite as soft and cooked as I was used to and it was covered in several kinds of seeds that I had never seen before. With my curiosity spiked to level one hundred, it did not take long before I asked my colleague about it. It turned out it was a raw dehydrated bagel.

I said: "What is that? A raw what?" It was the very first time in my life that I had seen anything like it. That was all it took, and my questions started pouring out of me like water out of a tap.

I soon found out that my co-worker's friend was studying to be a holistic nutritionist and she had made that bagel the day before as an experiment. It truly was the most amazing thing I had ever seen. My brain could not even begin to imagine how something like that could be made.

As the days passed by, I could not take that bagel out of my mind. It was not about the shape or flavor or anything like that. It was about the beyond-the-fact message that the bagel had sent me. I finally had proof that there was something more out there, something outside of my bubble that I did not know about. There was the hope of a better way, the hope that perhaps if I changed my lifestyle, I would have a chance to get out of the deep hole I was in.

The mysterious idea of the bagel never left me. It was like a seed that someone planted in the deepest corners of my being. It was rooted, and it wasn't going anywhere. I decided to keep digging further and look for water to bring it to life. I decided to do everything I could to meet this person who knew something I didn't. I had a strong pull in my heart, a knowing that this would be the beginning of something new, that this was my way out of the bubble.

Today, this person, whom I had the immense pleasure to meet a little while after eating her bagel, is one of my closest and dearest friends. I am so grateful to her for showing up in my life the way she did. I am so grateful that she decided to make that bagel that day. She truly was the one who pointed me to the door of my bubble and the one who years later gave me the key to my final escape. Laura Luis from *PuraEco Integral Wellness* is and always will be my greatest source of inspiration and a role model I will be eternally grateful for.

The key message in this beautiful chapter in my life is that when you get clear on what you want, and you keep looking for it in everything that shows up, you will eventually find it. It's not a matter of "if" but "when."

If you are looking to get over an illness, get curious about it and read everything you can on the topic. If you are looking to lose weight, find someone who did it and model yourself after them. If you are looking to learn how to prepare healthy meals, start shopping at health stores, read health magazines, and join whatever blog or group that draws your attention. Staying at home and feeling sorry for yourself for having failed in the past is not the answer.

BE OPEN TO NEW POSSIBILITIES

As soon as you become aware of the limitations of your perceived reality, you will become bombarded with new ideas, new thoughts, and new experiences that you may not be used to. They may feel strange and will not always make sense to you. It is imperative to stay rooted and not allow yourself to get overwhelmed. As per the raw bagel example above, I could have chosen to be scared of it. Instead, I just accepted that it was something outside of my known environment, something that was coming my way to help me expand and grow. I did not understand it, and I did not judge it. I allowed the idea of a new way of eating to flow into my life without interfering. I watched and observed with curiosity and openness.

Many ideas about getting healthy can seem overwhelming. Not surprisingly, the thought of letting go of our favorite foods, or following a new exercise routine, can be really scary for many of us. Of course they are! They are things outside of our comfort zone. We have no reference to them, and we simply don't understand them. Or worse, sometimes we may link them with some negative prior experience. Take a green smoothie, for example. I met so many people who at the first site of it rejected it immediately, having assumed that it would taste like the boring green salad they ate not too long ago. Whatever negative association they had with its color or texture limited them from being able to experience it fully.

Being able to see the limiting environment in which you have lived all along gives you a unique advantage. It allows you to understand why you are who you are today. Every decision you ever took in the area of your health has been based on the availability of ideas, thoughts, beliefs, and references that you have been programmed with in your past.

The great news is that you can begin to escape your limiting environment by borrowing ideas, thoughts, and beliefs from others to help you expand your own space of awareness. The key to being able to activate this process lies in your ability to see your own limitations and to be open to new possibilities even though you may not understand them. When you are open to discovering a new way of doing things and when you advance in life with curiosity, what you need will come your way, guaranteed. Awareness will dissipate the fog in front of your eyes, clarity will point you towards the door, and curiosity will turn the key in the latch. Together, all three are you way out of your bubble.

Chapter 2.4

LIVE FROM THE END, AS IF YOU ALREADY HAVE IT

Never mind what is. Imagine it the way you want it to be so that your vibration is a match to your desire. When your vibration is a match to your desire, all things in your experience will gravitate to meet that match every time.

−ABRAHAM-HICKS

Everything we create in our lives starts with a thought. Close your eyes and imagine for a second that being healthy is truly possible; that even though you may not know how right now, there is a way and you are committed to finding it. Feel what it would be like to have an abundance of energy. Imagine what it would be like to feel unstoppable, strong, clear, focused, and truly alive. What would you be able to do if you felt that way? What would your days be like?

When a problem seems too overwhelming, we often just freeze and do nothing about it. As Mark Twain once said, "The secret to getting ahead is getting started." The key is to take that very first step and to celebrate every bit of progress. Believe that you will get to where you want to be even if you don't know how.

The way to get started is first to imagine what it would feel like to already have that which you desire. Remember the example I gave you with my stepdaughter's wish of having a specific toy gecko? She had never seen it before yet she was able to describe it to me in great detail. And guess what? It took me more than two months of online searches to find exactly what she wanted, and in the end, I did it. I found the fuzzy green gecko that she imagined with googly eyes, a twisted tail, sticky toes, and yellow spots on its back. In a strange and inexplicable way, she knew she was going to have that toy before we even knew it existed.

You see, when you start getting clear on what you want, and you imagine having or being that which you desire, the universe conspires to bring it to you. Whether it is the law of attraction popularized by the famous book *The Secret* or a sacred alignment of energy as often described by the late Wayne Dyer, whatever it is, I can tell you something. It works! Think about it. Do you have something today that once was a mere thought, something out of the ordinary perhaps?

In the 1990s I was a young adolescent in Romania, just about to complete my last year of high school. One of our teachers asked us to write a note in the yearbook about a dream we desired to come true by the ten-year reunion. Though I had no idea at the time, or any prospects of ever studying or living abroad, what I wrote in that book was a desire that in ten years I was going to return home for the high school reunion on a plane. I was going to live so far away that flying would be the only way to get home. I saw myself buying the ticket, going to the airport, getting on that plane, and awaiting with anticipation the several hours that it would take to arrive at my destination. It was less than a month from that day that I received in the mail a letter of invitation to attend university in a small town outside of Toronto, Canada. The rest was history. And yes, I did fly home for my high-school reunion.

Coincidence or not, only this universe truly knows. What I do know and wholeheartedly believe is that when you get really clear on what you want, when you become truly open to the possibility of your heath goals coming to fruition, and when you use curiosity to get past any fears you may have, the universe will conspire in inexplicable ways to support you and keep you on the path to living the lifestyle you desire and deserve.

STEP 2 – Key Takeaways

1. Begin to switch your attention from your outer self to your inner self. Do so by always asking questions such as:
   a. How do I feel about this?
   b. Does this make sense to me?
   c. What do I really want?
   d. What are my mind, body, and soul telling me?
2. Move from constantly focusing on "doing" to just "being." This is a shift from what you have to do to live your life, be happy or solve a problem, to how you need to be in order to achieve the same. It's about letting go of the need to control everything and just allow nature to take its course. This is the true secret to feeling peaceful, relaxed, and worry-free.
3. Start getting curious about what you are afraid of. Ask questions about it, research it, and look at it from all angles. The more you find out about it, the less intimidating it will become. Knowledge is power. The more you know about it, the less power it has over you.
4. Start paying attention to new and unfamiliar thoughts, ideas, and objects that come to you from your inner or outer environment. The more open you are to change, the more of these will show up. Don't be afraid of them. Stay open and curious to everything that will unfold.

Recommended Reading: *As a Man Thinketh* by James Allen

STEP 3

BUILD A STRONG FOUNDATION

Chapter 3.1

OPTIMUM HEALTH REDEFINED

Most people have no idea of how good their body is designed to feel.

—KEVIN TRUDEAU

I know that you probably can't wait to get started and find the secrets and strategies for achieving optimum health. And trust me, I cannot wait to share with you all that I have learned and experienced over the years. The best moments of my life are when I see a new client experience for the very first time what optimum health and energy feel like, that inexplicable feeling of sheer light, clarity, and unlimited strength. It's as if you awake for the first time after a long period of sleep. What you thought felt great pales in comparison. What you thought you were able to do before is nothing but a dim light in the face of a new and powerful star. I have heard so many people say that they have never felt so alive, so awake, so 'themselves.' They are in awe of this total sense of peace and clarity that takes over when their body is allowed and supported to become the best that it can be.

Our body is our temple, the tool we were given to express ourselves into this world. It is a vehicle that carries out the orders we give it and allows us to carry out our mission. As with any vehicle, the better you take care of it, the better it will run and the farther it will take you. To do so, it is not enough to just know the strategies and shortcuts. Knowing something is not enough to get you to build a sustainable, healthy lifestyle. Information is everywhere in thousands of books, blogs, and websites on health and nutrition and in the words of so many so-called 'experts' that claim to know the latest shortcut to losing weight and changing your life.

You have to get to a point where you know what optimum health really is, a point where you understand it, you breathe it, and you live it!

Sadly, misinformation about what health is has been sabotaging people's progress more than bad food itself. Few things are more painful for me than seeing my clients build invisible walls on their paths to optimum health because of what they believe to be true or not in the area of health and nutrition. Whether it is because of the media, our educational system, our culture, religion, and even our parents' beliefs, most often than not, the notion of being healthy has been so twisted and polluted that its true meaning has been lost. Depending whom you ask, being healthy is about not smoking, not drinking, not consuming fried foods, working out, taking vitamins or having a salad every once in a while.

As you will see, I did all of that, and I still did not feel my very best. I always felt there was something missing. My heart and my soul whispered to me that I could be more and do more. Today, several years later, after a radical shift in my lifestyle and my choices, health has a completely new meaning for me. It is not about being vegan, vegetarian, or fruitarian. It is much more than the mere absence of disease and injury. Rather, it is about feeding my body with the most nutritious and high-quality food there is. It is about feeding my mind with empowering thoughts and feeding my soul with love and joy. It is about allowing my body to work its magic to heal me and to provide me with a relentless energy that radiates from every cell in my body.

This incredible force is hidden dormant in most of us because we are not giving our body what it needs to activate it. It is like a seed left to die in a dried-out, lifeless soil. But give it water, give it nutrition, and give it some light, and this seed can grow into the most majestic of plants.

One of the best ways to make life-long changes is to find someone that can support you and hold you accountable along the way. This can be a friend, a co-worker who joins you on your journey or a coach. When you work with a coach, for example, you are not left on your own to figure things out. Rather you have someone to hold you accountable, provide direction, and answer any questions you may have along the way. A coach is a teacher who will help you learn and understand how to choose healthy foods, how to prepare them in a way that protects their invaluable nutrition, or how to detoxify easily and safely. Whatever approach you opt to follow, remember to focus on learning and to understand the processes and tools you are given. One of the reasons many people don't get the results they desire from dieting is because they are simply following someone else's guidelines without internalizing this knowledge. A 'copy and paste' type approach will not give you long lasting results. If it did, diets would work for everyone.

The best way to learn something new is to immerse yourself in the process completely and to strive to understand and internalize the process, the tools, and the strategies. This way you can use the newly acquired knowledge to carry it forward into the future and be able to handle this area of your life on your own. My personal goal with all my clients is to empower them with all that is required for them to become independent, resourceful and confident in their ability to handle their health. A coach's goal should not be to make people dependent on them. It should be to pass on their wisdom to them and then let them grow and flourish in their own way.

I recently completed a six months health and wellness program with a lovely couple that asked me to help them take their health to the next level. Michelle and Dan had been regular customers at our restaurant, and so I had a chance to talk to them often about their goals and their dreams. Neither of them had any major health concerns, but for the last few years, they had observed many of their family members suffer from debilitating diseases, some even fatal. They were determined to do something about it but felt powerless in the face of the overwhelming and often contradictory world of nutrition.

As we started working together, I began, as I always do, to paint a picture of what was possible for them when they embarked on a new lifestyle focused on plant-based nourishment, juice cleanses, superfoods and highly energizing foods. Though nothing I said was beyond their ability to understand cognitively, it seemed though as if I was speaking in a foreign language. Dan, in particular, was utterly speechless when I spoke to him of not being hungry during juice fasts or the possibility of feeling so great some day that he would no longer need cigarettes to fill that void.

As the first day of the juice fast was quickly approaching, I could feel both of them becoming increasingly worried and excited at the same time. Despite their nervousness, I could see in their eyes a glitter of hope and a spark of determination to get through this no matter what. I do have to say that out of all the people I ever worked with, taking Michelle and Dan through the 5-day juicing program was by far one of the most memorable and magical of all such journeys. Michelle, in particular, suffered from severe detoxification symptoms and was on the brink of giving it all up. But she didn't. She followed through, and her efforts really paid off in the days to come. I will never forget the moment I saw them at the end of the five days. I will never forget the look of total joy and aliveness I saw on their face as they both described how they had never felt so great in their entire life. "Now I finally understand what you mean," said Michelle. "I can never go back to how I used to live because I now know the truth," she followed.

It is this 'truth,' this 'knowing' that I have the sincere hope for you to experience some day. The tools and strategies that you can use to achieve just that will be described in the chapters to come. Before we get there, we need to go over one last barrier that is standing in the way. We need to shine some light on several health-related myths that have steered so many people onto the wrong path. While I could spend the rest of the book going over all the misinformation out there, I have chosen to focus on six health myths that I found to be most prevalent and damaging.

Chapter 3.2

THE SIX HEALTH MYTHS TO LET GO OF

The best diet is not always the diet which is the best diet physically, but it's the diet that you can turn into a lifestyle that allows you to lose fat and keep it off because you learn how to incorporate all foods in healthy moderation.

—DR. LAYNE NORTON

One of the reasons diets and short-term strategies don't work is that they are designed for one to follow them without helping one truly understand how they work or how the body works to adapt to the changes suggested. So many people out there get on the diet train just to find themselves at the end of the program going back to their old ways. It is because they have not learned how to handle their challenge. They followed a set of instructions for a while and when the program was done, so was their progress. After studying over 150 different dietary theories, the only one way that I know to support long-term success is to learn and understand how your body works, how to help and support it, and to adopt new healthy habits and rituals that will stay with you forever.

Going over the following health-related myths will help clarify a lot of misinformation that has polluted the world of health and wellness over the last decade.

MYTH 1:
THERE IS A SHORTCUT TO GETTING HEALTHY

FACTS:
- *Quick shortcuts do not bring long-lasting results.*

- *Think consistent long-term results rather than short-term ups and downs.*
- *Quick strategies like taking weight loss pills or starting extreme fitness programs that promise major weight loss in short periods of time are just problem 'patches,' not solutions.*

I cannot even begin to tell you how many people have reached out to me asking for the latest and fastest strategy for taking charge of their health challenges in the least amount of time, whether that was losing weight, getting fit, or getting over some chronic illness. My answer to them is always the same: "you have come to the wrong place." What I do and what I teach is not about shortcuts; it is about empowering you with knowledge of all that is optimum health (i.e. mind, body, and soul) and supporting you in building healthy daily habits that will allow you to convert that knowledge into a sustainable lifestyle. Short-term quick patches simply do not work in the long term.

While it is true that life today moves at a much faster pace than ever before, the area of your health is not something you can rush. It may have taken you years to get to where you are today; that is not something you can just delete and start over. Your body needs time to heal and reverse years or months of damage. For some of you, it may take as little as a few weeks or months and for some a couple of years. Whatever your circumstances are, know that once you do start applying the right strategies and you follow them consistently, *you will* get results and *you will* once again be in control.

The best way to get started is to stop waiting for the "quick patch" solution to come your way and to focus on the very first step or action that you can do. Small actions taken consistently over time will yield great long-term results.

Getting healthy is not about popping the next super weight-loss pill, drastically reducing calories consumed, or jumping from zero into the latest insane fitness program. Rather it's about slowly adding more and more healthy habits to your daily routine that, in time, will bring big changes in your life. The law of compounding, though most often used in financial terms, applies in this case as well. The more small changes you add on top of each other, the more momentum you will get and the faster you will see results. Just breathe, relax, and take it one day, one step, and one new healthy habit at a time.

MYTH 2:
TO GET HEALTHY, I HAVE TO GO ON A DIET

FACTS

- *Traci Mann, UCLA associate professor of psychology and her co-authors, conducted the most comprehensive rigorous analysis of 31 diet studies. According to Mann, "You can initially lose 5 to 10 percent of your weight on any number of diets, but then the weight comes back."*[1]
- *Diets can be alienating, stressful, and depressing.*
- *Diets suggest you need to be deprived of something – not a sustainable strategy.*
- *Diets are not aligned with all that is unique about you (i.e. biochemistry, genes, blood type, metabolic type, etc.); therefore, one thing will not work for everyone.*
- *Diets don't take lifestyle and individuality into consideration.*
- *Diet food is not always nutritious food.*

This is not to say that diets don't work at all. Some do, but more often than not it is a game of luck as we are not all the same and no one thing will work for everyone in the same way. Many diets focus on reducing or eliminating certain macronutrients from your meals, such as carbs, fats or protein. Others require time to calculate either the right amount of calories or the right amount of ratio between proteins, carbs, and other meal components. You tend to spend more time trying to figure out what you 'should' do instead of actually doing it.

After studying over 150 dietary theories and having a chance to see them all in practice, I discovered that what might work for me, may not work for you, and the other way around. While I choose to follow a mainly raw vegan diet, I am always aware that such a lifestyle may not work for everyone. Thus, to reach your health goals, you must switch your focus from following the latest fad diet to learning the universal laws of optimum health and to apply them in a way that works for your unique self.

There is one more thing I would like to mention, one big misconception that needs to be clarified once and for all. Almost everyone I know who ever had a weight problem used the diet approach to resolve it. Let's get clear on something: weight gain is much more than just an issue of choosing one diet program over another. Weight gain is often a consequence of not living in your optimum health zone; it is an issue of consuming too many acid-forming foods, a result of inflammation, stress or being unhappy. So if you truly want to lose weight and keep it off forever, immediately change your focus from dieting to getting healthy. When you reach your optimum health zone, when your body works the way it should, weight will come off on its own.

To be able to reach this zone, it is imperative that you discover and begin to apply what I call the *universal laws of optimum health*. These laws will help you no matter where you are in your life and what goals you have. That's because they focus on one thing and one thing only: to provide your body with all that it needs to work as it should be. These laws include the need for maximum nutrition, hydration, cleansing, alkalizing, stress management, and movement. All of these have a direct impact on your body's ability to build and sustain a high level of energy and vitality, which in turn will support you on your journey to optimum health. In the chapters to follow, we will go into depth into each one of these, with specific examples for applying them in your daily life.

MYTH 3:
GETTING HEALTHY IS ALL ABOUT CUTTING CALORIES AND LOSING WEIGHT

FACTS:
- *Not all calories are made equal (i.e. calories from sugar are not the same as calories from greens).[2]*
- *Empty calories starve your body.*
- *You need optimum nutrition (i.e. healthy calories) to achieve balance.*
- *Weight gain is not the problem; it is a symptom.*
- *Losing weight quickly is unhealthy and may result in further weight gain in the future.*
- *Most rapid weight loss is water loss, not fat loss.*
- *Losing weight is about eating more...more of the "right" things.*
- *To lose weight you have to eat more fat...the "right" fat.*

Over the course of the last decade, I've had the privilege to work with many people all over the world looking to improve their health. This allowed me to identify many of the patterns and traps that people fall into in their quest to take their lifestyles to the next level.

One of the most common goals that people have is that of losing weight. The challenge is that, more often than not, people either are not clear as to why they want it or are completely overwhelmed and confused due to the amount of contradictory information out there.

Is that your story?

Do you feel like you've tried everything and nothing worked?

While it is true that weight loss plays an integral part of a good health and wellness program, the way it is accomplished makes a world of difference.

Maintaining a healthy balance between calories consumed versus calories used is an important strategy for losing and maintaining your weight. Even more important is to change your focus from cutting calories to choosing quality calories.[3] For example, avocados and cashews, though high in calories, provide you with essential nutrients that your body needs to thrive. These include Omega 3 fats for improved cognitive function, monounsaturated fats that can reduce bad cholesterol, and magnesium, which plays a major role in maintaining healthy skeletal and cardiovascular system.[4] In contrast, calories from simple carbohydrates (i.e. sugar, sweets, white bread, white pasta, white rice, etc.) are "empty" calories with a low nutrient value, which cause you to eat more and have less energy and health in the long term.[5]

Aside from some medical conditions, which cause weight gain and require specific strategies to be dealt with, most weight gain is caused by an acid-alkaline imbalance. When you eat too many acid-forming foods, your body will tend to store fat as a way of protecting itself in its struggle to remain slightly alkaline. When you start consuming foods high in alkalinity, your body will naturally let go of most fat deposits, as they will no longer be required as a buffer against acidity.[6] More on this will follow in Chapter 4, as we will go into more depth on the topic of alkalinity and its relationship to optimum health.

The key message to remember is to always focus on your journey and not the destination itself. When we become obsessed with losing weight, we often tend to make the wrong choices in an attempt to get there faster. Instead, slow down, steadily apply the techniques presented in this book and enjoy every bit of progress.

MYTH 4:
BEING HEALTHY MEANS BEING FIT

FACTS:
- *While being fit has tremendous benefits in oxygen creation and detoxification, it does not address the issue of lack of micronutrients and other essential components of a healthy regimen.*
- *Exercising in an anaerobic way most of the time can cause the body to be even more acidic and thus reduce the positive effects of working out.*

A client named Julia recently came to me to help her figure out why she felt tired all the time. Julia explained that she was an amateur runner and believed she was leading a fairly healthy lifestyle. At first glance over her health history checklist, she appeared to be doing quite well as her regimen included high-protein vegetarian meals, regular fitness routines, supplements, and a relatively balanced diet. But appearances can be misleading. As we started working together, the underlining issues came out. The base upon which she was building her life was weak and threatening to collapse at any time. She was exercising regularly outside of her target heart rate, which caused increased acidity in her body due to the build-up of lactic acid. She was also consuming high amounts of processed fats and drinking highly contaminated water. Over time this had weakened her body's ability to digest and absorb nutrients properly. As a result, she was highly anemic and severely dehydrated. It was only after cleansing, hydrating, and nourishing her body, that she regained her strength and was able to continue with her training in a healthy and sustainable way.

On August 15, 2015, Scott Ellis was riding in his nineteenth bike race in the Colorado Mountains when he collapsed unexpectedly. He soon after passed away with the cause of death being cardiac arrest due to significant atherosclerosis. He had major heart disease that he never knew of. Scott was 55. Too young to have heart disease, wouldn't you say? And he was fit, so how could this be? He exercised regularly, felt like his health was good, tried to eat right, and saw his doctor on a regular basis.

Sadly, Scott's example is one of many athletes who have passed in similar ways due to illnesses that they never knew they had. When you are fit and active, there is a somewhat false sense that all is okay. In reality, that is not always the case. The key to a healthy lifestyle is to work *with* your body and not to overexert it. Pursue fitness as an integral part of your lifestyle and include highly nourishing foods, proper hydration, regular detoxing programs as well as strategies for a balanced mind and spirit.

MYTH 5:
SWITCHING TO A VEGAN/VEGETARIAN DIET WILL MAKE ME HEALTHY

FACTS:
- *Vegan or vegetarian food is not all made equal; some can be highly processed junk food that can cause more harm than good.*
- *Many vegan or vegetarian diets are missing key nutrients that are essential for a healthy body and mind.*

To eat or not to eat, that is the question!

I can't even begin to tell you how many people have asked me what exactly I was eating now that I became a 'vegan.' From giggles and comments about eating 'rabbit food' to concerns over being protein-deprived or empathy for eating tasteless food, I have heard it all. "So what do you eat exactly?" they ask. "Don't you get tired of salads all day long?"

The answer is simple. Being vegan or vegetarian has nothing to do with being healthy or not. It's just a term designed to showcase your food category choices, and that's about it. Over the years, I have seen and read about many people following a vegan diet who got sick as a result. And I have also seen many, myself included, for whom making the shift saved their lives.

As I have emphasized before, the focus needn't be on the type of food you put in your mouth. Instead, focus on the quality and quantity of it. If you consume processed, deep fried, and highly acidic vegan or vegetarian foods, you are bound to get sick eventually. A lot of junk vegan and vegetarian food these days is marketed as healthy. Examples include low-fat foods, fat-free foods, processed gluten-free foods, high-sugar beverages like bottled fruit juice, vitamin water, etc. Rule of thumb: If the product ingredient list includes something you cannot identify, then it is probably not good for you. Remember always to read the labels and look for high-quality and clean ingredients. If you can't read it and it does not sound like food, then it most likely isn't food.

To wrap this up, I do want to make something very clear. Vegan or vegetarian food can taste amazing. You don't have to sacrifice flavor when eliminating animal products from your diet.

I will never forget the day when I met my current life partner. David was a trained chef with many years of experience and quite a few culinary wins under his belt. He was also a top-to-bottom 100% carnivore who could never imagine a life without meat, mostly because of his cultural background and because the one thing his culinary training emphasized more than anything else was the use of animal fat to get the best flavor.

I had not seen him for a few years and when we finally reconnected we were on completely different paths in regards to our lifestyles. I was shopping at local farmers markets looking for the freshest green leafy vegetables, and he had recently filled his freezer by purchasing something along the lines of half a cow. Let's just say that our first dinner together was quite interesting.

The most amazing thing happened when he first noticed the satisfaction with which I was enjoying my meal made of vegetables and seeds. The last time he had seen me I was sneaking into our company's kitchen to grab one of the meatballs he had just prepared for a catering event. He simply could not imagine that I was no longer craving meat or fat, nor needing them to enjoy food.

As the days passed, David joined me in writing my first raw vegan cookbook and slowly but surely things started to change. The first time he tried my vegan cashew cheese sauce, he was in awe. By the time we got to the raw desserts, he was pretty much sold. In all his years he had never tried anything like it. And guess what? There was no meat...there was no dairy. It did not take long for him to join me on the same path. The result of this incredible journey was the birth of one of the healthiest organic vegetarian restaurants in Toronto, Canada. *Thrive Organic Kitchen and Café* is a dream come true for both of us; it is our way to show the world that vegetarian foods are not just amazingly good for you; they can also be full of flavor and yummy goodness. Many of our clients are regular meat-eaters who understand the importance and the role that clean, nutritious, and easy-to-digest vegetarian food plays as part of a healthy lifestyle.

MYTH 6:
EATING GLUTEN-FREE IS GOING TO MAKE YOU HEALTHIER

FACTS:
- *Except for severe allergies (e.g. celiac disease) and intolerances, gluten can represent a good component of one's regimen when consumed in moderation.*
- *Gluten-free products can be highly processed and acidic.*
- *Gluten-free diets can be harmful to healthy gut bacteria. Rice flour, cooked potato flour and starch, tapioca flour, corn meal, and most other gluten-free flours or starches are poor sources of prebiotic fiber.*
- *Gluten-free diets may cause weight gain due to the use of many highly refined starches and simple sugars.*

In all my years working with clients looking to improve their health, I have yet to encounter a topic that is more baffling and misinterpreted than a gluten-free diet. Twenty years ago, when I began my career in the food service industry, you never heard of such a thing as a gluten intolerance or allergy. Today, two out of every five clients visiting our vegetarian restaurant are looking for gluten-free options, and health stores are packed with countless snacks, foods, beverages, and even supplements.

Many people switch to a gluten-free diet thinking that it is healthier. That may be true for some, but it solely depends on the quality of foods you are choosing. Often, gluten-free versions of traditional wheat-based foods are actually junk foods and thus can be even more harmful to your health. Many gluten-free products contain ingredients such as rice starch, cornstarch, tapioca starch, and potato starch, which are used as replacements for flour containing gluten. These are highly refined carbohydrates, and often release more sugar into the bloodstream than the original foods containing wheat. These can raise insulin levels and cause inflammation.

Gluten is a natural compound of certain grains like wheat, spelt and rye. It both nourishes plant embryos during germination and later affects the elasticity of dough, which in turn affects the chewiness of baked products. The real issue behind gluten intolerances is not the presence of gluten itself; it is the number of gluten-containing products we consume. In moderation, gluten-containing foods can form a healthy part of a balanced diet without causing any harm. Remember always to choose *whole foods* that naturally contain gluten such as Kamut, spelt, barley, etc., and avoid highly processed foods or foods that had gluten added to the ingredients list.

Here are some examples of wonderful gluten-free alternatives for those choosing to eliminate or reduce gluten intake:

- Grains/Seeds: quinoa, millet, buckwheat, amaranth
- Bread made with the grains/seeds mentioned above as well as chia and/or flax seeds
- Raw wraps made with either coconut meat or a mix of flax seeds and vegetables
- Noodles made with buckwheat, black rice, and/or sweet potato
- Raw seed and veggie crackers
- Sprouted legumes such as chickpeas and mung beans

Examples of ingredients found in many highly processed gluten-free products that you want to avoid:

- White rice flour – highly processed, low nutrition, simple sugar
- Tapioca flour – has a very high carbohydrate and caloric content; if you are trying to lose weight, this may not be the best food to add to your diet
- Cornstarch – highly processed, often GMO, raises insulin and causes inflammation
- Potato starch – highly processed, often GMO, raises insulin and causes inflammation
- Potato flour – simple sugar, raises insulin
- Cane sugar – often highly processed
- Canola oil – highly processed, often GMO, increases inflammation
- Vinegar – highly acidic unless it is apple cider vinegar

- Xanthan gum – produced by bacterial fermentation of a sugar-containing medium, which is often a potentially allergenic substance such as corn, soy, or dairy

Whether you choose to eat gluten-free or not, the key point to remember is that optimum health will not come from the types of foods you choose. It will come from their quality and nutrient availability. Always aim to purchase and use whole foods as much as possible and check the labels for added sugars and preservatives.

As you will learn in the chapters to come, the journey towards optimum health is about going back to our roots and applying some of the universal health laws that have been with us since the beginning of time. We have forgotten how amazing it is to feel fully energized, empowered, and unstoppable. Our bodies and our minds are sources of power that when expressed can take our lives to unlimited heights.

When you learn to align your lifestyle to the eternal health-related truths, you will not need to pay attention to the latest fads in nutrition, weight loss, and health in general. The only thing you will need to listen to is your body which, in its innate wisdom, will send you the exact clues and messages you need to hear in order to heal yourself from the inside out.

STEP 3 – Key Takeaways

1. Health is much more than the mere absence of disease. It is a hidden force of energy hidden in all of us that deeply impacts our mind-body-soul connection and thus forms the base upon which our whole lives are built.
2. There is no shortcut to getting healthy. Your health challenges were not created in a few days. Avoid shortcuts and let your body take its time to heal.
3. Most diets are shortcuts, quick fix attempts that may cause more damage long-term. Forget diets and focus on making long-term lifestyle changes.
4. Focusing solely on calorie counting, weight loss or getting fit is not sufficient to help you reclaim your optimum health.
5. Despite popular belief, vegan, vegetarian and gluten-free foods are not always aligned with good health. As you will soon find out, not all foods are created equal.

Recommended Reading: *Wheat Belly* by William Davis, M.D.

STEP 4

PLAY TO WIN – PICK THE STRATEGIES THAT WORK FOR YOU

Chapter 4.1

TREAT THE CAUSE, NOT THE SYMPTOMS. YOUR LIFESTYLE IS YOUR MEDICINE!

If all you do is treat symptoms, you are not going to cure the disease.

What you need to do is change the root cause.

—DR. DAN ROGERS

- What would your life be like with an abundance of energy and vitality?
- What foods are best to eat to help your body detox?
- What clogs your system and how is that impacting your life?

Welcome to the next stage of your life, ladies, and gentlemen. This is finally the moment where the tire meets the road, where we are permanently out of the bubble and ready to take on some new, empowering actions.

At this point, we can no longer deny that there is something out there greater than who we think we are, greater than the limitations of the confined space we had spent our time in for so long. We can no longer deny the fact that our physical body, the systems by which it works, as well as the invisible force of energy that permeates through every single cell, can be taken to a whole new level of existence.

So get ready and pay attention, as what I am about to share with you today has the power to create a major shift in your life and health. If you don't remember anything else I said, do read and remember this, as these are unique health and wellness secrets that your doctors may never share with you, not because they wouldn't want to, but because they simply have not been trained to do so.

Remember, my goal is not to overwhelm you with more information. Rather, it is about empowering you to create a clear road map from where you are today to where you want to be using strategies that work for you and your unique self.

Earlier on I shared with you, my story of growing up in a family where everyone suffered from all kinds of ailments. From depression to cancer, from heart disease to constipation and high cholesterol, I had seen it all. Having a pharmacist and several doctors in my own family, pills, creams, and other concoctions never seem to lack. They were everywhere – a pill for this, another pill for that, a never-ending array of drugs that surrounded me everywhere. I remember vividly every trip to the doctor's office and how I was always amazed as to how they remembered the names of hundreds of drugs and how they knew to match them with an illness so quickly.

One thing always crossed my mind, one question that they often were not able to answer. *Why?* Why did we get sick? What caused all those symptoms?

In these questions, my friends, rests the real secret!

You see, traditional medicine (a.k.a. Western medicine or Allopathic medicine) most of the time focuses on suppressing symptoms rather than identifying the root cause and eliminating it. Thousands of drugs had been invented to address every symptom and a small few to cure the cause. For example, if you have Type 2 Diabetes, your doctor trained in Western medicine is most likely going to prescribe medications for increasing insulin and balancing blood sugar. And then, to make things worse, you may end up taking other medications to address the myriad of side effects such as drugs for reducing cholesterol or triglycerides.[7]

So what if instead of taking all these drugs, we simply asked the question *why*? What if we looked for *the cause* instead of suppressing the symptoms? Well, if we did that, we would most likely find that one of the biggest causes of Type 2 Diabetes are poor diets filled with bad fats, highly processed ingredients, and acid-forming foods like dairy and other animal products.[8]

When you remove the cause, the problem is gone forever. When you treat your symptoms only, you are doing nothing but covering up the real problem. It's like trying to get rid of weeds in your garden. No matter how many times you cut them, they grow back, faster and bigger than before. You have to pull out the roots in the same way that you have to pull the roots of any health imbalance if you truly want to reach your optimum health zone.

Start listening to your body for signals that it is sending you in the shape of what we call "symptoms." Whatever you may be suffering from (e.g. headaches, arthritis, constipation, depression, diabetes, etc.), start asking: "Why? What made me sick?" Question anything that does not make sense to you and don't take it for granted just because someone who appears to be an expert told you to. While traditional medicine does have its place and is often very much needed to deal with some genetic diseases and bodily injuries, most chronic illnesses can be addressed with a holistic approach focused on total body healing (i.e. mind, body, and soul).

THE UNIVERSAL LAWS OF OPTIMUM HEALTH

You can't keep one disease and heal two others. When the body heals, it heals everything.

—CHARLOTTE GERSON

Over the course of my career, I have read hundreds of books on the topic of nutrition, and more often than not, many of them were contradicting one another. Also, new and exciting diets, weight loss programs, and other fads for dealing with some aspect of your health show up out of nowhere like mushrooms after the rain. For someone who is especially new at this, the world of nutrition can be quite intimidating and overwhelming.

My goal and purpose of this book, as already described, is to make this as simple as possible and to open the door for you to a new world of possibilities. This is about inspiring you and giving you a jumpstart for setting things into motion. The more comfortable you get with the new techniques, routines, and foods, the easier the process will become.

I would also like to clarify that nowhere in this book have I ever used an idea, tool, or strategy without having tested it first. Every single principle described has been applied and evaluated by my clients and myself. Anyone can come up with ideas and concepts, but I believe none is proven until used and understood by those who teach it.

As mentioned in previous chapters, despite the fact that we are all different when it comes to our biochemistry, our genes, our blood type, etc., there are some things that we all have in common. This is what I call the *universal laws of optimum health*. To put it in another way, this simply means that no matter what health challenges you may have, no matter how small or big they are, no matter what age you are, what genetic tendencies you have, these universal principles are crucial for you to master in order to allow your body to function at its best. There are many such laws that govern our health but for the purpose of this book and keeping in line with the idea that less is more, I have chosen to focus on six laws that I feel would give you the boost you need to take your life and health to the next level.

They are as following:
1. The law of optimum hydration
2. The law of maximum nutrition
3. The law of balanced alkalinity
4. The law of detoxification
5. The law of movement
6. The law of stress management

When mastered and followed consistently, these laws have unbelievable power. They lay the foundation of health and give your body the canvas it needs to "activate and reactivate its healing mechanism," so beautifully described by Charlotte Gerson in the documentary *The Gerson Miracle*. Whether you are healthy or sick, these laws must be a constant part of your lifestyle as they will either help you stay healthy or help you build the road to recovery.

As you read the following pages, remember that the journey to optimum health is not about achieving some ideal state of perfectionism. Rather it is about creating healthy habits and sticking with them. It is about preventing what can be prevented and healing what can be healed. And beyond all that, it is about living with joy and fulfillment on your terms, not anyone else's.

THE MEAT OR NO MEAT DILEMMA

Before we dig into all the good stuff, I'd like to take a moment and share my thoughts with you on the consumption of animal products and the recommendations I make in this book.

While I do acknowledge the fact that some people choose to consume meat and dairy and have no health related consequences from doing so, my approach is to always offer you the most up to date information so that you can make the best decisions possible for you. Research regarding animal product consumption has been pointing out the negative effects of such diets more and more in recent years. During this year's American Medical Association conference held in Chicago, it was announced that "based on scientific study, all hospitals and medical institutions should not only start to offer plant-based foods in every facility but should also remove all meat, dairy and eggs from their menus."[9]

Every recommendation I make in this book will be based on the consumption of whole plant-based foods and the principle of maximizing your micronutrient intake. The focus will be on both raw and cooked foods with an emphasis on super-hydration, building cellular energy and sourcing the highest quality foods possible.

Chapter 4.2

LAW #1:
THE LAW OF OPTIMUM HYDRATION

Pure water is the world's first and foremost medicine.

—SLOVAKIAN PROVERB

When I began my journey a few years ago, drinking more water was one of the early health principles I was exposed to. I have to be honest with you that my first reaction was something along the lines of: "Seriously? Drinking more water? I already know this! I drink water all the time." Oh, my! Was I in for a major reality check!

Let me just say something before you jump onto thinking as I did. The idea of drinking more water is not the solution. It's not as much about quantity as it is about quality. Some of you may be surprised to hear that not all water is created equal. Most of us have no idea as to the true nature of water and the effects it has on our health. Water can have an incredible power to heal, but some can also cause harm when consumed on a regular basis.

TYPES OF WATER – BENEFITS AND CONCERNS

I remember as a little girl we once visited a beautiful retreat center in the middle of the Carpathian Mountains in Romania. It was filled with different natural springs coming from beneath the rocks. Each spring was numbered and identified to be completely different in mineral composition from one another. People would visit the wellness professionals, and instead of lists of chemically laden pills, all they would receive was a small piece of paper with some numbers on it. I found that fascinating. It was something along the lines of: 9 am: Spring #6, 11 am: Spring #8, 4 pm: Spring #2, etc. No matter what health concern you had, your prescription was just water, miraculous healing water.

Though I was just a little girl, I never forgot that experience. It is one of my earliest memories of the healing power of nature and probably the earliest seed implanted in my mind that caused me to question so many unnatural and artificial foods and healing techniques that I was exposed to later on. Ann Wigmore put this eloquently when she said: "The food you eat can be either the safest and most powerful form of medicine or the slowest form of poison."

As with food in general, all types of water fall into one of two categories: natural water (i.e. natural, direct from source, not processed in any way) and treated water (i.e. water that has in some way been filtered or altered through various processes). Our goal here is to make things simple so let's look at four types of water that you are most likely to encounter in your day-to-day life.

Tap Water

Tap water is your basic water that you have access to in your home or office. Every city can have a different filtration system, and while some are great, there are also many that can leave traces of bacteria, lead or chlorination by-products. Also, there is additional possible contamination that can occur from old pipes leaching in your home or apartment building. It saddens me to say that unfortunately, most tap water is not always safe water. I highly recommend that you have your water tested by a reputable agency and drastically reduce or eliminate the use of tap water for drinking. In addition, you can purchase shower filters to reduce the possible contaminants that enter your body. Some of the most popular ones out there are Culligan, Santevia and Aquasana. Do some research and choose the model that fits your needs and budget.

Purified and/or Alkalized Water

Nowadays there are thousands of filters and purifications systems out there, each one promising the best and cleanest water. Some ionize, some alkalize, some eliminate a wide range of toxins, and others demineralize and remineralize your water. So what is one to do? If you are truly interested in getting a water filtration system, then make sure you do your homework. Recent research points towards the benefits of using alkalized water, and while consumer reports are promising due to its proved aid in detoxification, there are also studies that have shown a high consumption of alkaline water to lower stomach acid. This can cause issues with B12 and protein absorption as well as lowered protection against bacteria entering the blood stream.[10]

The process of sorting through all these options can be daunting so let's make this quick and simple. Ionized and/or alkalized water is generally much better that tap water and so stick to that for lack of a better option. Get the best filtration system you can afford for your home and when you are out and about choose ionized or alkaline water in glass bottles. The good news is that there is a better alternative, which we shall talk about shortly.

Distilled Water

While distilled water has many applications and has been shown to assist in the process of detoxification, many believe it is not the best option for everyday use due to the lack of minerals. Distilled water can also be slightly more acidic than other types of water and, therefore, caution must be exercised if it is intended to be used long term. As with tap water or purified/alkalized water, this one also falls into the category of 'altered' water. Hence it is not in the original state designed by nature.

Spring Water

Natural mountain spring water is some of the healthiest water on the planet because it is "living water." It is in its raw, natural state the way nature intended. Remember to always purchase and store in glass bottles to avoid possible contamination from plastic materials and do your research to ensure the water has not been altered in any way.

Spring water can be found for sale in glass bottles in most health stores. Nowadays there are also many companies offering home or office delivery. Be extra-careful with those and do your homework. Request that they share with you information regarding its source, bottling process, and to disclose if it has been treated in any way. Depending on where you live, you may be lucky enough to find a local spring next to your home and thus get it for free. This is an excellent weekend activity to do as a family and enjoy this beautiful gift that nature has to offer. Check out the website www.findaspring.com to see what is available in your area.

HOW MUCH WATER SHOULD I DRINK?

The answer to this question depends on several factors such as your bio-individuality and lifestyle choices. In general, to keep it simple, drink half your body weight in ounces per day. For example, my weight is 120 lbs., and so I aim to drink about 60 ounces of water per day. You may need to drink more depending on the following situations:
- In hot or humid temperatures
- During exercise
- When consuming alcohol or coffee
  - Coffee is extremely dehydrating, and it can take up to a liter of water to combat the diuretic side effects of a cup of coffee
- When enjoying a sauna, steam room, or hot yoga class
- While hiking at high altitudes
- When experiencing an illness such as diarrhea, vomiting, or high fever
- When pregnant or breastfeeding

SUPERCHARGE YOUR WATER

If I had to pick only one universal law to master first above all else, it would be the law of hydration. Our body is comprised of approximately 70% water, which is absolutely essential for all internal processes to take place. Drinking a glass of water here and there is nowhere near enough to keep you hydrated.

There is also a big difference between drinking water and actually absorbing it. When you drink the wrong type of water as per our examples above, you may not absorb much of it because it may not contain the essential minerals, electrolytes, and salts to keep it in your system. These components of water are necessary for your body to absorb it and stay hydrated. As I already mentioned, natural mountain spring water contains many of the essential minerals that the body needs, which is why I highly recommend it to everyone.

In addition to choosing mountain spring water, there are a few other techniques I'd like to share with you that can supercharge your water and provide even of these magical ingredients. This is by far my favorite way to boost my energy throughout the day. So here are a few ideas that you can choose from on a daily basis:

- Add fresh lemon juice to your water, especially in the morning, to help alkalize your body (i.e. juice of half a lemon per 0.5 liters of water).
- Add a pinch or two of Himalayan salt or Celtic sea salt per liter of water to increase your body's ability to retain it.
- Add MSM (Methylsulfonylmethane) powder to your water. Start with a little (i.e. half teaspoon per liter) and increase until you find the perfect flavor balance for you. MSM can improve skin complexion, detoxify the body, strengthen nails and hair, accelerate healing, naturally increase energy, and protect against inflammation.[11]
- Add raw organic greens powder to your water. Supergreens products are typically made from grasses, green leafy vegetables and algae harvested at their peak nutritional state. They are dried at low temperatures to preserve their nutritional value thus making these a true powerhouse of nutrition.

Adding these simple ingredients to your water is such an easy thing to do. It takes no more than a couple minutes in the morning to prepare your water bottles for the day or to pack some of these to take with you for later use. This is one of the best ways I know to boost your energy and to properly hydrate and maximize your nutrient intake.

WHEN SHOULD I DRINK WATER?

The time and amount of water you drink can also have a significant impact on how you feel. Here are a few tips for getting the most out of drinking water:

- Your body is most acidic upon rising, so drink a large quantity of water (one liter or more) immediately after waking up. Here's a great tip: leave a large glass of water by your bedside before heading to sleep. This ensures you will not be late in starting your morning hydration ritual just in case you choose to spend a few extra minutes in bed.
- Sipping warm water every 10-15 minutes throughout the day helps to activate your lymphatic system and thus detoxifies your body. This is a great strategy to use as part of a cleansing program.
- Drink water at least 20 minutes before or after meals so as to not dilute the enzymes necessary to break down food.
- Do not wait to feel thirsty before you drink water; by then your body is already in a high state of dehydration.
- Make water-drinking a habit. Buy an environmentally safe water bottle and carry it with you everywhere. Glass or stainless steel bottles are the best choices. Avoid all plastic and aluminum bottles. It takes a bit of time to build a new habit, but before you know it you will make this an integral part of your new lifestyle and your body will thank you.

Drinking the right kind of water in the right quantity and at the right time is an essential requirement for optimum health. Critical systems in our body, such as the digestive system, circulation, and excretion, cannot function without it. Here are a few of the many health benefits you and your family will enjoy once you begin to implement the tools and strategies I shared:

- Healthy body weight
- Proper digestion and nutrient absorption
- Healthy, glowing skin
- Better sleep

- Reduced inflammation and toxicity
- Better circulation
- More energy

Recommended Reading: *Your Body's Many Cries for Water* by Dr. F. Batmanghelidj

Chapter 4.3

LAW #2:
THE LAW OF MAXIMUM NUTRITION

Our food should be our medicine, and our medicine should be our food.

–HIPPOCRATES

Out of all the things I learned in my journey, the following concepts helped me the most in getting over the old, limiting beliefs I had in the area of my health:

1. Being healthy is not just about eating less – *it is about eating more, more foods with as many nutrients as possible.*
2. Being healthy is not about eliminating fats – *it is about eating more fats, the right kind of fats.*
3. Being healthy is not about completely eliminating sweets from your life – *it is about enjoying the right sweets in moderation.*
4. Being healthy isn't just about eating clean, organic foods – *it is about getting to the next level of "superfood" nutrition.*

Let's look at these individually and understand how each of them will help you in maximizing your nutritional intake and in giving your body what it needs for optimum health.

1. HOW TO MAXIMIZE YOUR NUTRITIONAL INTAKE

A "micronutrient" is a substance that provides nourishment essential for growth and the maintenance of life such as vitamins, minerals, antioxidants, and phytochemicals. The more nutrients your food contains, the better your body's ability to maintain optimum health.[12] The number of nutrients in food does not depend solely on what it is (e.g. a tomato versus spinach versus bread). It also depends on how it was grown, transported, stored, and prepared for consumption. The following factors can have a huge impact on nutrient quality and density:

- The mineral composition of the soil it was grown in
- The time it was picked (i.e. ripe versus unripe)
- How it was transported from the source to your grocery store shelf and how long it was held on the shelf before you bought it
- How you prepared it (i.e. kept raw, steamed, grilled, deep fried, etc.)
- Whether you used oil or water in the cooking process
- Whether the food (e.g. nuts, seeds, etc.) was prepared in a way that increased its nutrient density (i.e. soaking and sprouting)
- Whether it was treated with pesticides or not
- Whether it was injected with growth hormones, such in the case of animal products and by-products (i.e. eggs, milk, cheese, etc.)

Based on the factors above, here are a few facts you must be aware of so that you are empowered to make the best decisions possible:

The Soil
The mineral composition of the soil in which food was grown has a tremendous impact on the quality of food you consume. Soil depleted of nutrients through overuse or by applying pesticides will produce food that may look the same on the outside, but on the inside, it would be weak and low in nutrients.

So how can you make better choices while keeping this in mind? It is nearly impossible to know this information unless you have your own garden and have the soil tested. While I am aware that this is not a reality for many of us, growing your own fruits and vegetables and picking them ripe just before consumption, is the best way to get all the essential nutrients your body needs.

Another great way to achieve the same is to shop at local farmer's markets when possible and to eat food that is in season. The higher the % of local and in-season food you consume, the tastier it will be and the better it will be for your health.

Distance and Time
Many fruits and vegetables today are being transported from one country to another and picked before they are ripe to ensure they survive the long trip from home. While it is nice to enjoy exotic fruit from faraway countries without having to fly there, it is just as important to consume as many local fruits as possible.

Every region in the world has its own selection of fruits and vegetables that provide the entire array of nutrients our bodies need. Produce picked locally is a lot closer to the ideal ripeness and, therefore, cannot be compared with something that traveled from miles away, picked too early and treated with gas and other technologies to ripen them artificially before they reach your local grocery store. Get to know your local farmer's markets, visit local pick-your-own farms, build your own garden or start simply by planting a few herbs in your windowsill. Learn to fall in love with real food all over again.

Heating and Cooking Foods vs. Soaking or Eating Raw
The process of heating food causes many of the enzyme and nutrients in it to be destroyed.[13] Hence, raw foods (i.e. food not heated above 118 Fahrenheit) are more nutritious, and you could benefit tremendously by ensuring they represent a minimum of 60% or more of your meals to start with and around 80% as a long-term goal.[14] It is also essential not to heat oils as through that process they can convert into toxic substances.[15] Except for oils with a high smoking point (i.e. coconut oil, avocado oil), all other oils should be added to your food after cooking. We shall discuss more on this in the upcoming section.

A great trick to increase the nutrient content of grains, nuts, seeds, and legumes is to soak or sprout them before use. These can be a bit rough on your stomach and digestion due to the fact that they contain enzyme inhibitors that prevent them from being digested well. The soaking process increases the availability of nutrients and helps eliminate these digestive inhibitors.[16] Roasted nuts and seeds, for example, have little to no nutritional value. You can still enjoy them as a savory snack by choosing raw dehydrated nuts and seeds from your local health store.

Recommended Reading: *The Blender Girl* by Tess Masters

Clean Food
By "clean food" I am not referring to the simple process of washing your veggies. I am also referring to the amount of pesticides and chemicals that are added to food for many reasons such as to extend their shelf life, to resist pests, or to increase their ability to survive transportation. Whatever the reason, always remember that looks can be deceiving. Get informed and don't take what you see for granted. Just because the label says it's healthy does not mean it is. Be curious and know every step of the way that what you put in your mouth is what you become. Your body regenerates every moment of every day, and the cells of your body become that which you feed them.

I remember when I first heard the term "organic" a few years ago. I was reading a new cookbook that emphasized the use of organic ingredients, meaning they had been grown or prepared without the use of chemicals and other toxic compounds. I thought to myself: "Wait a minute, isn't that the way food is supposed to be like to begin with?"

Growing up on my aunt's farm, we never had to worry about what was in our food. Everything came directly from nature without any alteration. Today, sadly, we live in a new reality. We can choose to deny it but it is not going anywhere. It is important to raise your awareness in this area so that you can make conscious choices in sourcing your food. You have just one life, and so you deserve the very best that nature has to offer.

Organic food can be found in many health stores, farmers markets and even in some of the bigger grocery stores. A great little trick to be able to identify organic produce is to check the small sticker that they are identified with. If the code on the sticker begins with a number 9, that means the fruit or vegetable in question is organic. This is your best choice. If it begins with a number 4, it means the product is 'conventional,' in other words, it has most likely been grown with the use of pesticides and fertilizers. If you choose to buy produce with this code, it is important to peel the skin prior to consumption. While this will help lower the amount of pesticides ingested, it will also lower your nutritional intake as most vitamins and minerals are located in the skin.

If it begins with a 3, the produce also falls in the 'conventional' category but it has most likely been irradiated. And lastly, if the code begins with a number 8, this means the product is genetically modified. It is the last two categories that you want to avoid.[17]

When visiting farmer's markets, this identification system may not be observed, and thus it is best to always speak with the farmer to get to know them and the methods by which they grow their food.

2. HOW TO CHOOSE THE RIGHT FATS

Research now shows that the amount and type of fats we consume can have a tremendous impact on the way we think and feel. Our bodies need fat for insulation, vitamin and mineral absorption, and to protect our organs. High-quality fats can balance our metabolism, keep hormone levels even, and nourish our skin, hair, and nails.

Some of the types of fats that our body needs include saturated and monounsaturated fats, cholesterol, Omega-3s, and Omega-6s. While the first three can be synthesized in the body, the Omega-3s and -6s need to be obtained from food.[18]

The most important thing for you to know is that not all fats are made equal. Heavily processed and hydrogenated "trans" fats used in many processed foods can be extremely damaging to the body. Also, saturated fats from meat and dairy products are clogging and can compromise the cardiovascular system, immune system, and contribute to behavior problems.[19] They can also lead to weight gain, skin breakouts, high blood pressure, and liver strain.[20]

Excellent sources of fat can be found in avocados, avocado oil, oil cured olives, cold-pressed extra-virgin olive oil, raw extra-virgin coconut oil, MCT oil (i.e. coconut oil derivative), raw whole nuts and seeds, raw nuts and seeds butter (i.e. almond butter, tahini, sunflower seed butter, pumpkin seed butter, etc.).

Here are a few tips for how to source and use healthy fats:
- Look for oils of the highest quality possible. Words to look for: raw, organic, first-pressed, cold-pressed, extra-virgin, and unrefined. Avoid expeller-pressed, refined, and solvent-extracted oils.
- For cooking at high temperatures try organic avocado oil or coconut oil.
- Oils that have a lower smoking point, like oils made from avocado, flax seed, sesame, walnut, and pumpkin seeds are best used unheated in raw sauces, dressings, or drizzled on food after cooking.
- Research on the use of olive oil is mixed. I personally never heat it, especially if it is the extra virgin type. Should you ever decide to use it for cooking, I highly recommend you keep the temperature to low or medium.
- Excellent sources of Omega-3 essential fats include fresh avocado, avocado oil, algae oil, flax seeds, flax seed oil, chia seeds, sacha inchi seeds, hemp seeds, hemp seed oil, walnuts, and dark leafy vegetables.
- Great sources of Omega-6 essential fats include sunflower seeds, pumpkin seeds, sesame seeds, borage oil, etc. Those who eat lots of vegetables, fruits, nuts, and seeds already get enough Omega-6 to be healthy. The trick is to make sure you are not consuming too much Omega-6 as that may inhibit Omega-3 absorption.[21]

Recommended Reading: *Optimum Nutrition for the Mind* by Patrick Holford

3. HOW TO CHOOSE THE RIGHT SWEETENER

Hmmm...what can be more delightful than the mesmerizing smell of a bubbling apple pie fresh out of the oven or the soothing aroma of freshly baked cookies?

Yummy! As you can tell, I have a sweet tooth myself. Don't let that fool you as sugar, in reality, is something I am very careful with. As I said before, not all sugar is made equal. Some types can be okay in moderation, and some need to be completely eliminated.

The challenge about sugar is that, even though you may be looking to avoid it, it often comes with different names and forms that help disguise it. This often makes it impossible to identify. Here are a few of the most common forms of sugar: dextrose, glucose, high-fructose corn syrup, lactose, aspartame, saccharin, sorbitol, mannitol, etc. In fact, there are over 50 different types of sugars.

So what is one to do? First, keep it simple. The more homemade foods you prepare from scratch, the more ability you have to control the amount of sugar you take in. Secondly, for all other purchases, get familiar with the different names of sugar and become like a hawk. Check every ingredient list and look for healthier substitutions. My rule of thumb always is that if I cannot recognize the ingredient, I simply choose to avoid it.

Fortunately, for all us with a sweet tooth, nature has provided us with some yummy and delicious alternatives that we can use in recipes or on their own. My favorite ones are raw honey, maple syrup, coconut nectar, and whole-leaf stevia extract. There are many other foods that can also be used as sweeteners such as dates, raisins, vegetables like sweet potatoes, or sweet fruits like bananas and mangoes.

As with any sugar, it is important to keep everything in balance. Just because it's good for you does not mean you can eat the whole jar. Start searching for hidden refined sugars in your foods, explore some new and tasty alternatives, and use sweet foods as a treat, not a staple food.

Recommended Reading: *The End of Diabetes* by Joel Fuhrman

4. HOW TO TURN ANY MEAL INTO A SUPERFOOD

Since leaving the corporate world and opening my own health and wellness company, I've made some amazing changes and leaps in my lifestyle and energy. At 36 years of age, I feel more vibrant and alive than I ever did in my whole life. Looking back at my journey I can safely say that getting to this point had nothing to do with dieting or deprivation. The secret, my friends, is not about what you take out. It is about what you *add* into your life and into foods. It's about learning how to eat clean, how to listen to your body, and how to give it what it needs to reach its optimum health zone. One of the greatest ways to accomplish just that is through the use of superfoods.

Before we begin, let's get clear on what the term "superfood" means.

You will often see this word used in marketing as a way of describing foods with certain benefits, but that does not tell the whole story. In reality, a superfood is much more than that. It is a food item that contains very high levels of micronutrients in comparison to other foods. For example, some estimate Camu Camu berries as having thirty times more vitamin C than oranges and thus being the fruit with the highest vitamin C content in the world.[22] While it is not necessary to consume such high doses on a regular basis, having some Camu Camu on hand makes a world of difference for stopping a cold in its tracks.

I don't know about you, but I love chocolate. I eat it every day without exception. Not just because it tastes great but also because it is actually good for you. Yes, you heard me right! It is good for you! No, wait, it is not just good for you; it is *amazing* for you! Raw organic cacao contains a higher concentration of antioxidants than any food in the world.[23] I know that right now you are probably wondering: "How about blueberries or red wine?" Guess what? Raw organic cacao has more antioxidants by weight than both of them combined.[24] Isn't that amazing? The key to remember is that not all chocolate is made equal. Often it is highly processed, depleted of nutrients by heating to high temperatures, and laden with chemicals for flavor enhancement or preservation. Your best bet is always to buy raw organic chocolate that contains 75% or more cacao and is made with healthier sources of sweeteners such as raw organic cane sugar, coconut sugar, coconut nectar, or raw honey.

Other examples of superfoods include spirulina, goji berries, all bee products, aloe vera, hemp seeds, maca powder, moringa leaf powder, etc. You can use these in smoothies, dressings, sauces, desserts, and so much more. While I could spend the rest of the book talking about superfoods and how fantastic they are for your health, I could never do it justice, as could the God of all superfoods, David Avocado Wolfe. I wholeheartedly believe that his book 'Superfoods,' is a must read for everyone serious about mastering their health.

As you can see, healthy eating is not always about cutting something out. It is about how we source, prepare and consume food in a way that maximizes its energy, nutrition, ability to be digested and absorbed and thus get us closer to optimum health. It's about eating more, more of the right things! Here are a few examples for choosing the best foods in regards to quality and nutrition.

CHOOSE:
- Organic sourdough bread made with simple ingredients: organic flour, starter (fermented culture of flour + water), Himalayan salt, and spring water
- Raw sprouted seed bread
- Whole grains
- Organic, local fruits and vegetables
- Sprouted nuts and seeds
- Sprouted or soaked legumes (e.g. chickpeas, black beans, etc.)
- Fresh, raw, cold-pressed organic green juices
- Raw, dark chocolate made with raw, organic cacao
- Raw crackers
- Spring water
- Himalayan or Celtic sea salt
- Raw honey, coconut nectar
- Raw extra-virgin coconut oil or avocado oil for high heat cooking
- Cold-pressed extra-virgin olive oil, hemp seed oil, flax seed oil, borage oil, etc. for dressings

AVOID or DRASTICALLY REDUCE
- Bread made with preservatives, sugar, eggs, artificial supplements or GMO ingredients.
- Gluten-free products made with simple sugars and artificial ingredients
- GMO fruits and vegetables
- Dried or roasted nuts and seeds
- Simple starches (i.e. white flour, pasta, white rice, etc.)
- Bottled juices made from concentrate

- Animal products and by-products
- Milk chocolate
- Coffee
- Alcohol
- Deep-fried chips and other processed snacks
- Tap water
- Table salt
- Cane sugar, artificial sweeteners
- Vegetable oils (i.e. canola, sunflower, corn, safflower)

Recommended Reading: *Superfoods* by David Wolfe

THE IKEA CINNAMON BUN – AN ADDICTION CURE STORY

Have you ever had one of those cravings that no matter what you did, you could not get rid of? One of those delightful foods that you knew with utmost certainty would bring you happiness in the worst of circumstances? The kind that you would not stop eating no matter what anyone said?

I surely did!

Let me just say that the famous IKEA cinnamon bun was "it" for me. I mean, honest to goodness, it felt like this thing had complete control of me. You'd tell me that we were going shopping at IKEA and my eyes would light up, my heart rate would go up, my mouth would start salivating, and before you knew it, I was dressed up and ready to go. Nothing could stop me. Well, nothing other than the long line-up I had to go through before being able to bite into the ewwy-gooey double splash of icing that, without fail, I always asked the server for. And wait! That is not all! I would ask for two; two ewwy-gooey gigantic cinnamon buns that filled my soul and my belly with utter delight.

So you may be wondering what this has to do with anything. Well, it has everything to do with everything! This thing had total control over me for one good reason. My imagination. Yes, you heard me right. My imagination!

Aside from the fact that I had no idea what this magical cinnamon bun was made of, I would take this addictive ball of yumminess and turn it into the most irresistible drop-down gorgeous piece of dessert that you could ever imagine. I did all of that without any magical powers; I did it all in my imagination. I took something I already liked and turned it into a totally and completely irresistible product by simply altering my view it in my imagination. I mean I was a true movie producer and added real life sounds, smells, and special effects to this seemingly innocent piece of cake. I made it into a superstar! Don't we all seem to do that sometimes? We do. We do it all the time. We imagine a meal or food item being a thousand times more than what it really is, especially when we are really hungry. And that could actually be a good thing except when it is applied to something that does not serve us.

The way out of this is easier than you might think. It is not about giving up something you enjoy; rather, it is about knowing without a shadow of a doubt that you deserve the best, it is about raising your standards and looking at the challenge from a different angle.

While trying to come up with a solution to this, I asked myself the following questions: "What if I didn't have to give it up completely? What if I could change it to something that was actually good for me?" The result of this process was the creation of a simple three-step system that without fail allows me to make healthier choices in every situation. Here is how you can use my "Reinvent It" technique to improve the quality and nutritional availability of any recipe:

THE RE-INVENT IT TECHNIQUE

>STEP 1: Get clear on why love it and find what's in it.
>STEP 2: Recreate what's a must.
>STEP 3: Re-imagine it.

Here's what I mean. Think of a food item that you feel you must have and stop for a second to question whether it is good for you or not. I never believe in consuming foods that are tasteless and boring just because they are good for you. If you are lucky enough to find something that tastes great and also supports your health, then by all means, go for it (in moderation of course). But if the item you thought of is far from helping you get better, there is still an option available.

The first step is to get very specific as to what exactly you love about it. In my case, for example, it was not everything about the cinnamon bun that I loved or had to have. Once I slowed down and thought about it, I realized that what I loved most was the cinnamon flavor, the sweetness, and the texture combination of something smooth and silky (i.e. frosting) with something that had a bit of a bite to it (the bun). Once I got clear on that, I started doing some online research for similar recipes that met my musts.

That took me to step #2 where I recreated the recipe based on some new techniques I learned from my research. I decided to use baked apples to replace the bun as the texture was quite similar. Instead of the processed, sugar-laden frosting, I made a raw coconut nectar cashew sauce that was simply to die for. Let me just say that the IKEA cinnamon bun today pales in comparison to my new creation. A few sprinkles of cinnamon and some crumbled nuts and cranberries transformed this traditional recipe into something memorable.

Once I was happy with the flavor, it was all downhill from there. If I ever found my way shopping at IKEA, instead of using my imagination to turn the cinnamon bun into the latest superstar, I did the same for my super-duper apple creation. And guess what? When I got home, it took me less than ten minutes to recreate the same sublime experience. No feeling of deprivation, no flavor compromise, and no regret for consuming something that was not aligned with my new values of health and well-being.

And that, ladies and gentleman, is how I declared victory over my cinnamon bun addiction. Since then I have applied the same technique over and over again to different foods with the same lasting results. Remember, it's not always about cutting something out; instead, think a bit outside of the box and give that food a chance by reinventing it in a way that supports your health goals.

Chapter 4.4

LAW #3:
THE LAW OF BALANCED ALKALINITY

No disease, including cancer, can exist in an alkaline environment.

−DR. OTTO WARBURG,
1931 Nobel Prize Winner for cancer discovery

The pH balance measures the ratio of acidity and alkalinity in your body, which should be around 7.35, with blood and most tissues being slightly alkaline and urine or saliva being slightly more acidic.[25] Maintaining a proper ratio between acid and alkaline foods in your diet is crucial for your body to be able to maintain this number in a way that does not deplete your bones and tissues of deeply needed nutrients.

Without getting too scientific, the most important idea to understand is that your body is constantly working to maintain this crucial balance the same way that it maintains your heart pumping and your temperature at the exact level required to keep you alive. Every single thing that you put in your mouth will cause a response from your body, which will do whatever is needed in order to maintain this balance. For this to be achieved, your meals should be made up of 60-80% alkaline foods. If you are looking to maintain a good health, than you may be ok in the 60-70% range, but if you are suffering from an illness, it is recommended to get closer to the 80% range.[26]

Take a look below and get some sense as to the pH level of different products.

Acidic Foods (pH of 5 to 6.9 or less)
- All dairy and eggs
- All meats, cold cuts, and seafood
- Carbonated water, club soda, energy drinks, most purified water, bottled juices and pop, alcohol, coffee, black teas
- Honey, maple syrup, all forms of sugar, processed sweeteners
- Roasted nuts and seeds
- Dried fruits
- Refined grains and grain products (e.g. white pasta, bread, rice, etc.)
- Processed oils (i.e. margarine, trans fats, refined vegetable oils)
- Most cooked vegetables and overcooked grains
- Table salt
- Vinegar (with the exception of apple cider vinegar)
- All processed foods (i.e. jams, soy sauce, ketchup, mayonnaise, mustard, processed soy products etc.)

Neutral (pH of 7)
- Most spring water
- Most tap water

Alkaline Foods (pH of approx. 7-10)
- All fresh raw vegetables
    - Some of the top picks include spinach, collard greens, summer black radish, alfalfa grass, barley grass, cucumber, kale, jicama, wheat grass, broccoli, oregano, garlic, ginger, green beans, endive, cabbage, celery, and red beets
- All fresh raw fruits
    - Some of the top picks include citrus, dates, raisins, grapefruit, tomatoes, avocado, watermelon, figs, and ripe bananas
- All sprouts
- All legumes (soaked and/or sprouted is best)
- Some nuts and seeds (i.e. chia seeds, almonds, flaxseeds, sesame seeds, brazil nuts)

- Cold pressed oils (i.e. flax seed oil, hemp seed oil, raw coconut oil, extra virgin cold-pressed olive oil etc.)
- Some grains (i.e. quinoa, amaranth, buckwheat, wild rice)
- Seaweed
- Himalayan salt

You may be looking at this and thinking: "Oh my goodness, does this mean I cannot eat anything from the acid forming side anymore?" No, no, no! Not at all! It simply means that we need to eat in a balanced way that allows the body to safely maintain the appropriate pH level without having to resort to unhealthy means of achieving the same. When we consume too many acid-forming foods, our body must borrow nutrients from our bones and tissues to help maintain this fragile balance, thus affecting all other systems and our ability to stay healthy overall.[27] You can observe pH fluctuations in your body quite easily by purchasing some pH strips from your local health store and testing your urine fifteen to twenty minute after your meal. Test your urine three to four times daily for about a week to ten days and come up with the average. That will give you a great indication as to where you stand in general.

An example of an acid-forming meal would be a bowl of chili with bread. It may be organic, and it may be cooked the proper way, but if consumed on its own without a large green salad on the side, it would cause more acid to be formed in your body. To achieve the most optimal ratio, you can enjoy the chili with a large bowl of salad and skip the bread. Does this make sense? Here are a few more examples of balanced meals to help you out:

1. A large bowl of salad, a side of steamed veggies, and your choice of nuts or seeds. Nuts and seeds are best soaked to make them easier to digest. You can eat them as they are or prepare them into a nut and seed pate, dehydrated crackers, or dressings.
2. A large bowl of salad, a side of steamed veggies, and sprouted chickpeas or a mix of sprouted legumes. You can eat the sprouted legumes as they are or prepare them into a hummus-style spread.
3. Raw, sprouted seed bread with avocado, freshly sliced cucumbers, tomatoes, and Celtic sea salt.

4. A smoothie made with avocado, mixed berries, dates, spinach, kale, and some fresh coconut water.
5. A bowl of vegetable soup with a large side of lightly steamed veggies drizzled with flax seed oil and fresh lemon juice.

One of the most powerful ways to alkalize your system is to eat raw green vegetables with any meal, whether you are having breakfast, a snack, or your dinner. There are hundreds of recipes that you can experiment with by doing a simple Google search for alkalizing or raw vegan meal ideas. Keep in mind that overcooking your greens can also make them acidic. Consume them raw as much as possible or lightly cook them via steaming or water sautéing.

The second most powerful way is to regularly drink fresh green juices or spring water with fresh lemon juice and MSM powder added to it. Stay away from any bottled drinks and switch to making your own by investing in a juicer or simply using more and more lemon juice with your water and meals. Also, make a list of every single juice bar in your town, so you have a quick option for when you are out and about.

Switching to a plant-based alkaline way of eating was truly the catalyst that brought about the greatest shift in my lifestyle. Given the right environment, your body knows exactly what to do to keep you healthy, and an alkaline environment is exactly the place you want to be.

Set yourself up for success by printing the food list above and placing it in your kitchen or even save it to your phone for use when shopping or eating out. Whether you start with one alkalizing meal per day or go full out, know that you are on your way to taking your health to a whole new level. Challenge yourself a little every day and get ready to feel amazing!

Recommended Reading: *The pH Miracle* by Robert and Shelley Young

Chapter 4.5

LAW #4:
THE LAW OF DETOXIFICATION

Detoxification works because it addresses the needs of individual cells, the smallest units of human life.

—PETER BENNETT, N.D.

I suffered from low iron anemia my whole life. I was pale, tired, and weak most of the time. I took iron pills and ate chicken liver and other meat products that were supposed to fix my problem. Despite all that, thirty years later my iron was still low, and no one was ever able to tell me why exactly this was happening. All I ever heard was that I was born that way and that there was nothing I could do to fix it other than ensuring I was taking my daily pills and weekly doze of animal organs. Yikes!

It took me one too many years, but at 31 years of age, I decided to take matters into my own hands. I was not sure it was going to work, but I was ready to try something different. Going back to the old ways was no longer an option for me.

When I stopped eating animal products altogether, my family was terrified that I would become even more anemic. In my "common sense" mind, I couldn't imagine it was going to get any worse. I mean, my iron levels were a 3 on a scale that was supposed to range from 22 to 561 pmol/L. I was absolutely ready for trying something different. I stopped eating all meats, dairy, processed foods, fried foods, white flour and sugars, coffee, etc. and started eating a whole food, mostly raw, plant-based diet. It changed my life. In only two months I started feeling more energized and more alive than I ever did in my whole life. In only two months my iron level skyrocketed to levels it had never reached before.

I am not a doctor, but I know that I am my own expert. I know that if I were to continue listening to all those who apparently knew what was best for me, I would most likely still be stuffing myself with synthetic pills and daily portions of hormone-laden red meat.

My message is really quite simple. If you've tried something and it did not work, stop for a second and listen to your heart and your body. What are they telling you? Does your current strategy make sense or is it time for something radically different?

It turns out that the reason my body was able to heal when I switched to a vegan diet was that I had allowed it to do what it knows best. I provided it with the right foods that allowed it to cleanse and get rid of mucus and inflammation. After years and years of synthetic medicine and meat products, my digestive system was clogged and was not able to absorb anything. After allowing my body to cleanse and heal, it was finally able to absorb the nutrients I was giving it. All it needed was a timeout, a chance to detox and recharge.

Our body goes through the process of detoxifying all the time, every day and every night. It does so through our blood, liver, kidneys, lungs, lymph, digestion, and skin. Unfortunately, due to so much pollution, stress, and toxic food, our bodies are overwhelmed, and this amazing process is slowed down or altogether halted. Also, while some foods may seem to give us an energy boost (e.g. pastries, dairy, energy drinks, coffee), they actually deplete and clog our bodies and reduce the absorption of minerals and nutrients needed for optimum health.[28] It is our job to support the process of detoxification and give our body a chance to do what it knows best.

Here are some of my best tips and techniques that I have learned and used over the years and that have given my clients and me the ability to make a massive shift in our levels of energy and vitality.

IS A DETOX PROGRAM RIGHT FOR YOU?

New and exciting detoxification programs are coming out faster than we can keep up with them. There are herbal cleanses, raw food cleanses, fresh juice cleanses, fasting programs, etc. As with all things, not everything is created equal, so before you jump in, let's first understand what a detox program really is and when you should be doing it.

A detox program can help as follows:
- It gives your organs a chance to rest and rejuvenate
- It stimulates the liver and kidneys to drive out toxins from the body
- It promotes elimination through the intestines, kidneys, and skin
- It improves blood circulation
- It refuels the body with healthy nutrients

Here are a few signs you are in need of a detox:
- You feel *sluggish, tired, irritable*
- You experience *mood swings* or *difficulty concentrating*
- You feel *congested* or *bloated*
- You struggle with *digestive* or *skin* problems

If you do experience some or all of these on a regular basis, then it is time for you to give your body a hand. Whether you will choose to buy a herbal kit from the health store, do a raw juice cleanse, or do some other type of detox, ensure that you do your homework and avoid anything that does not make sense to you.

If you are new at this you may experience detoxification symptoms (i.e. headaches, fatigue, weakness, fever, etc.) due to the release of a higher concentration of toxins from your tissues into your blood stream. Sometimes it gets worse before it gets better. My recommendation is to not do this on your own. Instead, find a coach to guide you through the process and be with you step-by-step along the way. It is best to find someone who will show you the strategies and also teach you how to apply them so in the future you can handle everything on your own.

The good news is that you don't always have to take on complex detox programs to help your body out. Please see below a list of tips and strategies that you can add slowly to your daily and weekly rituals. The more you do, the better the results you will see.

Tips for Keeping Our Blood Clean:
- Drink lots of fresh live water (i.e. spring water and green juices), especially in the morning (see section on the law of hydration).
- Take chlorella supplements (i.e. powder mixed in water or tablets).
- Drink young coconut water – full of natural electrolytes that are critical to maintaining blood volume.
- Add fresh lemon juice, apple cider vinegar, MSM powder, or supercharged greens powder to your water to increase its alkalizing effects.

Tips for Keeping Our Lymph Working Properly:
The lymphatic system in our body is responsible for transporting toxins and waste products from your tissues so that they can be removed from your body.[29] Unlike the circulatory system, the lymphatic system does not have a pump to activate it and keep it working (the circulatory system is activated by the heart). Here are some of the best tips and strategies for supporting your lymph system and maximizing your energy:

- Rebounding is one if the easiest ways to activate the lymphatic system especially if you are a beginner in the world of exercise. Invest in a low-impact rebounder and enjoy it daily while watching TV or listening to music. Try it for 10-15 minutes twice a day for a week or so, and you will see your energy skyrocket. You can also enjoy jogging if you are more advanced or invest in a whole body vibration machine such as Hypervibe or Powercore.
- Schedule a lymphatic massage.
- Practice dry-brushing on a regular basis.
- Deep diaphragmatic breathing – see the upcoming section on lung support.

TIPS FOR KEEPING YOUR SKIN HEALTHY

About 60% of substances applied to our skin are absorbed, thus resulting in approximately 4.4 pounds (2 kilos) of chemicals every year entering your body.[30] Thus it is crucial to drastically reduce or eliminate unnecessary toxins from entering your body in order to allow it to function at its best.

- Remember that health on the outside is a result of health on the inside.
- Exfoliate:
    - Practice regular dry brushing.
    - Use wool gloves in the shower.
    - Exfoliate with natural bath salts.
- Cleanse and hydrate your face with homemade masks prepared with natural ingredients such as clay, avocado, lemon, honey, coconut oil, etc.
- Utilize healthy oils such as coconut or argan as natural body moisturizers instead of creams containing synthetic compounds.
- Use natural soaps, shampoos, body creams, and similar products that are plant-based (i.e. coconut oil, olive oil, almond oil, shea butter, etc.) with or without essential oils and herbs for scent.
- Avoid deodorants containing aluminum, triclosan, and other synthetic ingredients and look for natural varieties made with coconut oil, aloe vera, coconut oil, baking soda, and essential oils.
- Enjoy detoxifying baths with Epsom salts and essential oils like rosemary, eucalyptus, and lavender.
- Increase perspiration: allow your skin to sweat by going to the sauna, hot yoga, or steam room on a regular basis.
- Avoid toothpaste that contains fluoride, sweeteners, artificial flavorings, and colorings and instead, look for ones made with baking soda, coconut oil, and herbs and essential oils.
- For all you ladies out there, use sanitary pads instead of tampons and always buy natural, organic, unbleached and non-perfumed varieties.
- Install shower filters to reduce the amount of chlorine that comes in contact with your body.
- Practice hydrotherapy by alternating hot and cold water while taking a shower. First, allow your body to warm up in water that is as hot as you can handle. Then drop the temperature to as cold as

you can handle and hold for up to 30 seconds. Alternate two or three times for best results.
- As with anything else, avoid products that contain ingredients that you do not recognize. As I always say, never put anything ON your body that you wouldn't otherwise put IN your body.

TIPS FOR SUPPORTING LUNG FUNCTION

- Our respiratory system is one of the most important ones in the process of eliminating free radicals from our body. The fast pace of our lives, high-stress environments, improper posture, and a chronic lack of exercise all contribute to us not breathing in a way that allows our body to oxygenate properly and eliminate toxins.
- Practice deep diaphragmatic breathing several times daily to allow oxygen to circulate more deeply through your system (i.e. inhale deep into your diaphragm for 5 seconds, hold for 20 seconds and release slowly through your mouth for 10 seconds).
- Avoid highly polluted areas.
- If living in the city, walk in nature at least once a week.

TIPS FOR SUPPORTING LIVER AND KIDNEY FUNCTION

- Eat more bitter greens like mustard greens or dandelion; they can be juiced, steamed, lightly sautéed, or chopped and added to soups and stews.
- Drink freshly squeezed organic grapefruit juice.
- Eat foods high in vitamin C – this will help your liver increase the production of glutathione which helps drive away toxins (e.g. lemon juice, lime juice, Camu Camu powder added to smoothies)
- Enjoy teas made with dandelion root, burdock, and milk thistle.
- Take digestive bitters during spring or during a detox program.

TIPS FOR IMPROVING YOUR DIGESTIVE SYSTEM

- Hydrate: review section on the law of hydration.

- Maintain healthy gut flora by consuming fermented foods on a daily basis: coconut kefir, coconut water kefir, sauerkraut, kimchi, probiotics, fermented teas like kombucha or jung, etc.
- Increase fiber: whole fruits and veggies, chia seeds, flax seeds, etc.
- Eat heavier meals in the middle of the day so as to allow your digestive system to break them down before sleep; avoid heavy meals after 6 -7 pm.
- Enjoy fruits on an empty stomach always. Fruits digest very quickly and if eaten after a meal, they can cause severe bloating and fermentation.
- Consume lots of healthy fats
- Avoid processed sugars
- Benefits of colonics - colonics help cleanse the body of toxins by removing all loose fecal matter from the bowels. As with all things, moderation is key. Colonics can represent a wonderful tool to use during your annual detox regimen and benefits can be seen after only a couple of sessions.

Over the years, after completely revamping my lifestyle and working with so many clients on similar paths, I identified four key questions that allow me always to make the right choice when it comes to any meal. I call these my "4 to thrive."

1. Will it provide me with maximum nutrition?
2. Will it clog me or cleanse me?
3. Is this meal clean?
4. Will it make me more acid or alkaline?

These questions are entirely focused on maximizing your nutrition for optimum health. Next time you are about to make a choice for a meal, give this a try and see what a huge difference this will make.

Chapter 4.6

LAW #5:
THE LAW OF MOVEMENT

Those who think they have no time for exercise will sooner or later have to find time for illness.

—EDWARD STANLEY

My journey in the world of fitness and exercise was something along the lines of a roller-coaster ride. I didn't just wake up one morning to say: "Yay, I can't wait to go sweat for an hour and then have to go through two or three days of muscle pains." You know what I mean, right?

As with all other limitations, I soon realized that it was all in my head. Exercising was not something that was on the list of priorities for my family growing up or within the cultural and social groups I had been a part of.

After several attempts that did not give me the results I wanted, I realized I had to change my strategy. If I was going to excel in this area as I did in all the rest, I had to do something different. I had to change my strategy. And so, as we discussed in the early pages of this book, I started slowly, focusing on changing my beliefs about exercise and incorporating small step-by-step changes rather that going to an extreme. I chose not to overwhelm myself by making something bigger than what it needed to be.

Here are some of the best and most empowering questions and beliefs that I chose to focus on and that have helped my clients and me make major leaps in getting closer to our goals in the area of fitness.

POWER QUESTIONS:

- What is stopping you from working out regularly? What is the truth, not the fake story?
- What would you need to know or have in order to start taking action?
- What would you do first if you knew that or had that?
- What would you do second?
- Do you live to eat or do you eat to live?

POWER BELIEFS:

- Nothing tastes as great as being healthy feels.
- Today I commit to taking one more step towards achieving my fitness goals.
- I want and deserve the very best in regards to my fitness and level of energy.
- I love myself completely and take excellent care of my mind and body.
- I let go of all that I no longer need. My body is healing quickly and easily.
- My past is done, and I do not dwell on it. I live right now, in the present, with happiness, love, and joy.
- There is always a way if I am committed.
- I can use my creativity to take action and move forward; there is a fun way to get fit, and I will find it.
- I know this is a bit scary, but it is a million time scarier to imagine what the rest of my life would be like if I do not master this area now.

Aside from limitations stemming from your family's or social group's beliefs, routines, and priorities, another reason why you might dislike exercising may be because you had a negative experience in the past. Maybe you twisted your ankle, or maybe you worked out too hard, and you ended up in pain for a week. You somehow linked that one-time experience with a feeling that you do not enjoy exercising. The good news is that you can change that perspective if you are open to it. Imagine a time in your past when you actually had fun working out. Think about it in great detail and remember the feelings you had while doing so. Practice this remembrance as often as possible and as intensely as possible and it will help you greatly to begin to associate the idea of exercise to a positive experience rather than a negative one.

Just like detox programs, weight loss and fitness programs are popping up like mushrooms everywhere. Many of them promise you quick solutions without focusing on whether that is healthy and sustainable. I too fell for one of those a while back, before I had a chance to learn my lesson. Fast food may get you fast results but at what price? The same applies to exercise. If you want great and lasting results, you have to look for a strategy that works for you. Not everyone can run, not everyone can last for hours and hours of cardio, and not everyone can stand the heat of a Moksha yoga studio. The bottom line is that there are many options to work out and improve your fitness. Open your mind to the possibilities and look for something you love and have fun doing. That will ensure you will come back to it time and time again. Here is an example of a five-step exercise to help you in this process:

1. Rate the type of fitness programs below from 1 to 3 as follows:
   1 = "I really do not enjoy this type of exercise, and I do not see it as doable."
   2 = "I feel neutral about this, or it could go either way."
   3 = "I really think I can do this and I am open to giving it a try."
2. Evaluate all the ones labeled with a 3 and imagine yourself in the middle of that routine. Does it seem fun? Do you look forward to starting?
3. Pick two that are more appealing to you at this time.
4. Make it a must that in the next 48 hours you will take some action to show your commitment to giving one of these activities a shot. You can call a gym and make an appointment, you can make your commitment public with your friends on Facebook, your social group, or your family, or you can tell friends and ask them to help hold you accountable for taking action.

5. Write it on your calendar and commit to a time and day of the week when you will enjoy your new activity. Take it as seriously as you would any other appointment.

Here are a few examples to choose from:
- Rebounding (10-15 minutes twice daily)
- Brisk walks (20-30 minutes once or twice daily)
- Yoga
- Dancing
- Swimming
- Hiking
- Biking
- Tennis
- Rowing
- Jogging
- Join a team: basketball, soccer, badminton, etc.
- Join a gym that offers group classes like Zumba, cycling or aerobics
- Join a club that offers specialty classes such as Capoeira or Martial Arts

Whatever form of exercise you choose, here are a few key principles to remember:
- Exercising is not just about burning calories; it is about reducing stress and increasing oxygenation. This is why good aerobic exercise is so important for everyone. To achieve that, one should exercise within their ideal heart rate (one easy way to calculate is 180 minus your age)[31], which can be measured with a heart monitor or by watching your breath. If you can exercise and still carry a basic conversation with someone, you are okay.
- Rebounding is one of the easiest and fastest ways to increase your energy and oxygenate, and it is a particularly good form of exercise for beginners. Start with ten minutes once or twice a day and increase as you go along.

- Create an empowering environment in the area of physical well-being. Find a person or group of people that you can share the exercise with. This is by far the best way to get started, stay on track and make significant progress.

Chapter 4.7

LAW #6:
THE LAW OF STRESS MANAGEMENT

*Stress doesn't come from the facts.
Stress comes from the meaning we give those facts.
When we come up with a new meaning, we get: A New Life.*

—ANTHONY ROBBINS

Stress. What is it really? We hear about it in the media, in schools, at work, at home. It is everywhere, following us in our daily activities like our own shadow. In today's fast-paced environment, everything seems important, and everyone seems to want something from you (e.g. attention, time, money, etc.) We are in a constant go-go-go motion that increases our stress levels and affects our ability to cope with life's demands. Stress is one of the most serious problems of our time that affects us both emotionally and physically.[32]

    Writing this book was a phenomenal experiment for me. For the first time in a long time, I switched from doing to just being; I disconnected from the world and lived in my own space, just me, myself, and I. And the three of us had the time of our lives. No phone, no Internet, no appointments, no things to do other than writing this book and bringing the best of me to you.

    Finding a way to manage your stress is a crucial stepping-stone in building your health for success. Take a deep breath and think for a moment. Ask yourself: "Where does stress come from? Is it yours? Did someone give it to you or did you create it?" If you are true to yourself, you know that stress is something you create by either paying too much attention to something, making something bigger than it is or by creating imaginary and unrealistic scenarios to any given situation.

The good news is that, once we realize that we are the ones that create it, we can also escape from it. Here are a few key principles to assist you in this process:

- Get more sleep, rest, and relaxation - plan to go to bed and wake up at the same time every day and sleep in complete darkness.
- Get in touch with your spirituality - find ways to get in touch with your spiritual side, be it meditating, dancing, drawing, going to church or temple or being in nature, whatever works for you.
- Take time for yourself – engage in activities that restore your energy, such as a walk, a bath, a museum, a movie, or whatever you enjoy. Schedule a weekly date with yourself to do these things; make it a must, as nothing is more important than you.
- Create a form of regular exercise routine. Exercise has been proven to be one of the most powerful tools against stress.[33]
- Take five minutes every day to write down everything you are grateful for.
- Practice deep diaphragmatic breathing (see the section on detoxification techniques).
- Get rid of negative relationships. Some people can drain you of your energy and while they may not be doing it intentionally, this just means you are not aligned when it comes to your core values and beliefs. Spend time with people that support you and lift you up. See if you can transform those relationships by communicating and setting boundaries or end the relationship.
- Spend more time in nature.
- Focus more on what you *want* to do versus what you *have* to do.
- Practice letting go and responding to things as they come, rather than hypothesizing ahead of time of what may or may not happen. Thinking about the future creates stress, as we do not have control over it. All we can control is right now, so focus on the present moment and your next step only.

GROWING YOUNG

A few years ago when I was 26, I made a new friend who was just celebrating her 33rd birthday. One of the first things that struck me about her was how tired and exhausted she looked. It just never seemed to get better. One day I was complaining about feeling that way myself when she said the following to me: "You should not complain; you are just 26; wait till you are my age. Waking up tired, feeling sluggish, having wrinkles, dry skin, and bags underneath your eyes will be normal." What she said struck me so powerfully that I never forgot it. I just couldn't imagine my life like that.

Shortly after, my life took a new course, and I embarked on a new journey that took me in an entirely new direction. I changed everything about how I thought, felt, behaved, the way I made decisions, the way I ate, drank, and the way I took care of my body. The focus of my new lifestyle was about maximizing my energy, my vitality, my mental strength, and mental clarity. I ate better; I slept better, I was a brand-new me!

One day I remembered my friend and what she had told me and I smiled with tremendous pride and love for myself, and the force that guided me throughout this process. I smiled because in just a few months I was going to be 33 and I felt better and more alive than ever before. I felt younger, and I looked better than I did when I was 26. There was no magic trick, no mysterious pill or miracle diet. It was all that I shared with you in the pages of this book.

You now know the secrets of my success, and they can be yours, too. You now know the tools and strategies that I used for my clients and myself to build our health for success time and time again. Turn the power on inside of you and make a decision right now to turn your life around as well. Make it so powerfully that it becomes an absolute must; that no matter what may come your way, you will always put yourself first.

The better you are, the better everything else in your life will be!

STEP 4 – Key Takeaways

1. Find the real *cause* of whatever health challenge you may have, as that is the secret to getting rid of it forever.
2. It is *never* too late to reset your health no matter what anyone tells you. There is always something you can do to make it better.
3. To build a strong foundation of health, you must learn and implement the six universal laws for reaching your optimum health:
    - Optimum Hydration
        - Drink the best natural spring water possible.
    - Maximum Nutrition
        - Maximize the nutritional availability of your food by buying organic and local ingredients and using superfoods and healthy cooking techniques (i.e. raw meals, sprouting, dehydrating, low heat cooking).
    - Balanced Alkalinity
        - Help your body stay in balance by choosing 60-80% of your foods from the alkaline varieties.
    - Detoxification
        - Help your body detox by using different techniques such as juice fasting, rebounding, going to saunas, breathing exercises, etc.
        - Create your own cleansing schedule: daily, weekly, and seasonally.
    - Movement
        - Find something you love to do and do it as often as possible.
        - Treat your time to exercise as you would any other appointment.
        - If you feel like you do not have the time, make the time. Time is not something you "own;" it is something you create.
    - Stress Management

- Realize that stress is self-created and thus can be controlled.
- Find ways to manage and get rid of self-created negative stress to allow your body to heal.
- Some stress can be good for us as it can help us get things done, but research shows that negative stress can deeply affect one's health.

STEP 5

PULL THE ANCHOR AND LEARN TO HANG ON

Chapter 5.1

TAKE ACTION NOW

You are what you do, not what you say you'll do.

—CARL G. JUNG

So here you are, empowered with new tools and new knowledge and ready for your first serious commitment. I promise you that if you stayed with me so far, you have everything you need to take action and change your health and life forever. All you need to do is take that very first step, whatever it may be.

Are you going to join your first fitness class today? Are you going to go shopping at a health store for the first time? Or are you going to prepare and enjoy your very first green juice?

Whatever it is, remember that the most important thing is to focus on your first step only. Forget about tomorrow! Forget about next week! They are not real. What is real is the action that you are about to take right now. Stop building overwhelming stories about how you can't see yourself doing this for the rest of your life. Stop wondering how you will manage to pull this off with a big family and a full-time job. And for goodness' sake, stop thinking of the green monster juice and how awful you think it may taste.

Stop, delete, breathe, and just be and enjoy this moment for all that it has to offer you.

You are absolutely ready to take your first plunge. You know it's going to be a little painful at first, so don't fool yourself into saying that it won't. Just go with it. Take your fears, put them in your pocket, and leap together into the unknown. Do something, anything, no matter how small you may think it is.

One of these liberating plunges happened for me a few years ago when I attended my first personal development seminar. I had never done anything like that before because I had never made my personal well-being a priority. Somehow, the well-being of others seemed to be more important. So needless to say, I was terrified. I had just spent thousands of dollars on a promise with intangible results that may or may not come through. But I did what I had to do, pulled the anchors, and plunged. I took the annoying gremlins in the back of my head and stuffed them in my backpack. I told them that I was going on a trip and this place was way too exciting for them; too much music, too much fun, and way too many nice people.

Isn't it funny how sometimes we have no idea what is to come next, and yet we tend to build these overwhelming stories about what may or may not happen? We toss around worrisome thoughts about one hypothesis or another and wear ourselves to the ground, just to find out later that we had been completely out of line. Has that ever happened to you?

So here's a better strategy. Next time you are in a situation like this, let go, accept the truth that you have no idea as to how things will unfold, go with the flow, and when you finally see the result, respond accordingly. Try it, and I promise you that you will see a world of difference.

LET GO OF WHAT DOES NOT SERVE YOU

I will never forget the day I arrived back home after this life-altering experience. What I thought I knew about health, energy, well-being, and life, in general, was completely eradicated. I was in awe, inspired and full of curiosity just like the day I sampled my very first raw bagel.

I walked through the door of my house and got an instant feeling of being a total stranger in my own home. Objects like clothes and furniture didn't seem to belong; food items left in the kitchen caused me to experience a strange sense of sickness in the pit of my stomach. I simply could not imagine myself eating those foods ever again, foods that had been a part of my life since I was born.

In the days to come, I changed everything about my life. I threw everything out of my house, every synthetic piece of dishware, every ounce of processed and lifeless food, every toxic cosmetic and house-cleaning product. I threw everything out. I was no longer going to accept anything in my life that could potentially stop me or slow me down from growing into a higher version of myself.

I remember vividly sitting in the middle of my kitchen and watching the empty cupboards, counter, and fridge and imagining with anticipation the great changes that would come. Though I had no idea at the time how I was going to get all the things I needed for my brand-new lifestyle, I did not stop dreaming and envisioning my new space filled with life and energy-giving foods.

It is hard to describe in words the feeling of total freedom and liberation that I experienced. It was as if I had grown wings and taken flight for the first time in my life. To know and feel in every cell of your body that you and only you are in charge of what you will be and do for the rest of your life; that no one and nothing outside of you has the power to tell you that you are wrong or that you cannot do something. I wish that for all of you from the bottom of my heart!

Letting go of all that did not serve me was the beginning of a new chapter in my life. From that moment on I was going to be the one deciding what my body needed, not anyone or anything around me. Liberating myself from all that once defined me was absolutely necessary for me to be able to grow into the person I am today.

My sincere hope for you is that by the end of this book you will be just as inspired to take charge and make some major changes in your life. As I always say, this is your life, your only life, so choose healthy, choose happy, and do whatever you can to live always as the best version of yourself.

HITTING YOUR RESET BUTTON

In the days to come, I started bringing home fresh and exciting greens, herbs, and superfoods that would become an integral part of my first detox program. I bought my first juicer and with that began the first step of my new adventure. I was going to drink enough live and clean water and highly nutritious green juices until all that did not serve me in my body would be destroyed and eliminated. Juice after juice, I continued nourishing myself with all that I had been craving for so long. The feeling of complete euphoria and enthusiasm soon disappeared as the negative effects of detoxification started to show up.

Within just a couple of days, I was completely immobilized in bed with high fever and severe pains. I spent over a week lying in bed, fighting some of the worst symptoms I had ever experienced. Every day I'd wake up hoping this would be the day it would be all over, and then it wasn't.

As the days passed, I started to notice something changing. Alongside severe cold and hot sweats and uncontrollable cough, I started to notice my skin changing, my mind being quieter, my face getting brighter, and a feeling of peace and tranquility taking over. It was something I had never experienced before. And I knew right then and there that my life could not possibly be the same way again because I wasn't the same.

Something was changing.

Something was getting out of my body that did not belong there. And though it came in the form of pain, fever, chills, weakness, dizziness, and excruciating pain from all the coughing, it felt like a challenge, a test I had to pass to show I was truly committed. I wasn't going to stop. I wasn't going to give up. The strong feeling I had inside that there was another way to reverse illness and achieve optimum health grew stronger and stronger with each day that passed by.

At the end of just over two weeks, I woke up one day a brand-new woman. The feeling of utter exhaustion had disappeared; aches and pain were gone as if wiped out by an invisible force. I remember getting out of bed for the first time in a very long time with a renewed sense of energy and excitement. I ran to the mirror and right there in front of me was a brand-new person that I could not wait to meet. It was almost as if I had been gone on a journey back in time and was now getting to know myself for the very first time.

I had hit my reset button. I made it happen even though no one believed that I would.

Chapter 5.2

SET YOURSELF UP FOR SUCCESS

The road to success is not straight.
There is a curve called Failure,
a loop called Confusion,
speed bumps called Friends,
red lights called Enemies,
caution lights called Family.
You will have flat tires called Jobs,
but if you have a spare called Determination,
an engine called Perseverance,
a driver called Will Power,
you will make it to a place called Success!

—UNKNOWN

In Chapter 1 we took a quick glance at some of the factors in your external and internal environment that can severely affect your ability to achieve your health and wellness goals. It is time now to take a deeper dive into each one and share some tools and strategies for setting up an environment that will support you every step of the way.

WHO you spend time with is who you become
WHAT you spend time doing is who you become
WHERE you spend your time is who you become
HOW you spend your time is who you become

Everything in your surrounding environment affects you directly and indirectly: who you spend time with, what you have or do not have in your home, kitchen, washroom, or bedroom, how much time you spend in the house, where else you spend your time, how much TV you watch, how many books you read, how much you focus on educating yourself versus entertaining yourself, how much you eat out versus cook at home, how much you contribute to the well-being of others, how much you exercise, etc.

Whatever it is that you want to achieve, whether it is losing weight, healing a chronic illness, or completely revamping your lifestyle, you must always set yourself up for success. What does this mean? It means creating an empowering environment around you, an environment that supports you to succeed no matter what comes your way. Here are the four areas we are going to focus on at this stage:

1. Your peer group
2. Your home
3. Your access to healthy food
4. Your workplace

YOUR PEER GROUP

Your standards and your ability to meet your goals are highly influenced by the people you surround yourself with, whether that is your family, your friends, your co-workers, or people in social groups.

No matter how strong willed you are, if the people in your environment are not supportive of the changes you wish to make, eventually, you will lower your standards and go back to old habits. If you want to meet your health and wellness goals, it becomes essential for you to surround yourselves with people who play at the same level or higher. Here are a few key questions to help you identify possible limitations in this area:

- Is everyone in your family supportive of the change you wish to make?
- Are you friends supportive of the same?

- Are you surrounded by people who you can learn from and who push and support you to become more?
- Is there anyone that shares your values and passions?
- Is anyone overly concerned about the changes you are making and constantly sharing reasons as to why this may be dangerous for you?

Whenever you are in the process of making a change, open your eyes and ears as wide as you can and listen for any signs of anything that could potentially slow you down. If you are not sure whether someone would be supportive or not, it is best that you do not share your plans with them.

Here are a few examples of things you can do today to create a more supportive environment when it comes to the people you are surrounded with:

- Join a group with similar goals (i.e. a fitness club offering group classes, a sports team, a Facebook or Meetup group).
- Find an accountability buddy from any of these groups and support each other along the way.
- Get a coach or mentor.
- Volunteer in places where the focus is on health and wellness, like community centers or nonprofit organizations.
- If you have any friends that share similar goals, make it a must to schedule more time together (i.e. meet once a week for a healthy lunch or schedule a couple of short phone conversations a week to check in and see how each is doing).
- Get a part-time job at a local gym, health-oriented store, or restaurant.
- Let go of negative people; it is not your job to make them happy.
- Spend time with people who support you and love you.
- Don't try to get people to agree or understand what you are doing. Those who are ready to change will make themselves known. For the rest, just be the best role model that you can be.

YOUR HOME

The central philosophy behind all that I do and all that I teach my clients is that eating with a focus on maximum nutrition is absolutely essential to achieve optimum health. While that is unequivocally true, to stay healthy these days, we have to focus on more than just clean eating. We also have to consider minimizing our exposure to environmental toxins.

The British Medical Journal reported in 2004 that environmental and lifestyle factors are key determinants of disease in humans and that they account for about 75% of most cancers.[34] Studies show that women put an average of 168 different chemicals on their bodies each day.[35] Without making this too scientific, it is important to know that your skin is like a sponge and can very easily and quickly absorb whatever products you use. The great news is that there are many natural alternatives that you can enjoy without compromising your health.

Here are a few simple tips and strategies you can implement to minimize your toxicity exposure and help your body to work at its best.

Manage the air quality
- Avoid VOCs (chemicals that evaporate easily) in paint, carpeting, furniture, shower curtains, etc. Don't just buy something because it is cheap. Do your research and find out exactly what you are paying for.
- Whenever possible, stick to wooden floors, organic cotton, wool, or plant-based carpets, wooden furniture, paints with 'low' or 'zero' VOC levels, cotton or other plant-based drapes and shower curtains.
- Open the windows and air out your home every day.
- Use a wet diffuser with essential oils such as lavender and peppermint as air purifiers for your home, especially bedrooms and living rooms.
- Use a dry diffuser with essential oils such as clove, cinnamon, peppermint, or rosemary to help kill the mold in your home, especially in washrooms and basements.

- Replace regular paraffin or soy candles with 100% beeswax candles, which burn clean and release negative ions that help remove toxins from the air.
- Use Himalayan salt lamps to help keep the air clean, especially near computers, modems, TVs and other electronic equipment.
- Use plants to clean the air in your home (i.e. snake plant, peace lily, Boston fern, etc.).

Manage what comes in contact with your body
- Use shower and sink water filters to reduce chlorine and fluoride exposure.
- Wash your laundry with "soap nuts" (available at most health stores), baking soda or source 100% natural detergents from your local health store.
- Replace chemically laden dryer sheets with wool balls scented with your choice of essential oils (Geranium is one of my favorite ones).
- Learn how to make your own cosmetic or home-cleaning products or shop for clean and natural versions at your local health store or online. Avoid anything that contains ingredients you do not recognize.
- Choose 100% cotton (organic cotton is best) and other plant-based materials when shopping for bed sheets, lingerie, towels, and wash before first use.
- Implement a "no-shoes policy" in your home to reduce contamination from outdoor pesticides.

Design your special hiding spot
- Our homes can get quite busy and messy, especially when we have kids, a big family, and many visitors. Create a hiding spot where you can set things up the way you want without anyone disturbing them. It can be your office, a corner of your living room, or even your washroom. There are no rules other than making it your own and using it as a place to escape and be able to clear your thoughts and realign your mind, body, and soul with all that serves you.

For many of you, your home is your sacred place where you unwind, relax and let go. Make this a special place that supports you instead of hindering your progress. Keeping your home healthy and clean will help you tremendously on your journey towards optimum health!

Recommended Reading: *101 Natural Remedies* by Laurel Vukovic and Natural Health Magazine

YOUR ACCESS TO HEALTHY FOOD

I cannot emphasize enough how important access to clean and nutritious food is, as a tool for helping you reach your health and wellness goals. A supportive environment in this area includes the availability of health stores and organic products in the area where you live and work, the choice of restaurants and juice bars, as well as the food choices you have in your fridge, cupboards, and workplace. Here are some tips for setting yourself up for success by surrounding yourself with healthy choices whether you are at home, at work, shopping, or on vacation.

- Make a list of all the healthy places to eat in the areas of town where you spend your time, whether that is close to home, work, or a place you might be visiting; do some research online for raw, vegan, or organic food or look for a local vegetarian directory. Never leave home without a plan for eating.
- Avoid places that offer foods you have major cravings for while you are in the early stages of your change process.
- Never leave home hungry or go shopping hungry. The subconscious connections you have with food will make most of the decisions instead of your conscious mind. You want to be in charge, not your stomach.
- Always have healthy snacks and water with you, so you never let yourself get to a point where you feel like you are starving.
- Throw out all processed snacks from your home and replace with nourishing alternatives so if you are hungry or have a craving, you have better options to choose from. Having some dates or some

raw crackers with hummus is a thousand times better than choosing deep fried chips or cookies.
- Replace plastics and aluminum pans and containers made of stainless steel, cast iron, wood, paper, bamboo, and other natural materials.
- Invest in a good-quality juicer and blender, as these will allow you to exponentially increase the amount and variety of nourishing recipes that you will be able to produce (i.e. Omega, Huron, Norwalk, Vitamix, Blendtec, etc.)
- Invest in a nut milk bag to be able to quickly and easily prepare nut milk at home.
- Bring healthy snacks to work to have them ready to go just in case. This can include energy bars or a mix of raw nuts, seeds, dates, seaweed, etc.

Tips for making your cooking experience quick, easy and enjoyable:

- Pick a day of the week when you will be doing most of the prep work, especially for more complex items such as soups, stews, sauces, and dressings.
- One or two days prior to your "prepping" day, get organized:
    - Review your meals for the upcoming week.
    - Make a list of everything you need to buy.
    - Do all your shopping.
- Prep most veggies ahead of time:
    - Wash and cut vegetables and fruits needed for your daily juices and smoothies.
    - Buy prepackaged and washed lettuce greens (spinach, baby kale, arugula, mesclun greens, romaine, etc.) to save time.
- Freeze as many things as you can to have them ready to go when needed. Some great things that can be frozen are soups, stews, veggie patties, marinated broccoli and cauliflower pieces, diced squash or pumpkin, carrot fiber left over from juicing to be used in crackers, etc.
- If time is your concern, remember that healthy food actually takes less time to prepare. Meals cooked for hours and hours on end are

depleted of nutrients and will not serve you in the long term. A superfood smoothie will give you much more nutrition and energy than a heavy meat-and-potato stew, and it only takes five minutes to make.

YOUR WORKPLACE

When it comes to healthy eating at work, I think I have pretty much heard every excuse known to man.
"I do not have time to eat."
"There is no healthy restaurant around."
"I do not have time in the morning to prepare my meals."
I will be the first one to admit that I used to feel that way.

The first 15 years of my career in business were based in the food service industry, so needless to say I never had to worry about having access to food. But not all food is created equal, and sooner or later reality hit me. It became clear that I was not going to get any healthier by continuing to eat there. My only choice was to bring my own food. Easier said than done. Waking up early to prepare my meals was not something I ever had to worry about.

When something becomes a must though, somehow all these excuses seem to disappear. I started slowly, step-by-step, and made gradual changes without getting overwhelmed and frustrated. First, I started taking bottles of lemon water with me; then followed a few raw snacks here and there, and in a couple of weeks I started including one or two lunches. I never even realized how time flew by until one day I was preparing and bringing with me an entire day's worth of food.

No one says it is easy but if I could do it, so can you. Here are some of quick strategies and tips I learned along the way that you can start applying right away:

- **RESEARCH** - Do some research and make a list of healthy places to eat or source food while at work. If leaving the workplace is not an option, look for healthy restaurants that offer delivery or bring your own food.

- **PLAN** - If you will choose to make your food and bring to work, invest in some eco-friendly food storage containers to use on a daily basis. Avoid plastics and aluminum materials and, instead, choose containers made out of stainless steel, recycled paper, bamboo, and other natural materials. Your local health store is a great place to start looking.
- **TAKING FOOD TO WORK** - When taking food to work, avoid anything that needs to be reheated. That way you can avoid the harmful effects of using microwaves or the additional loss of nutrients. Here are some great ideas for lunches to bring to work:
    - Vegan nut and seed loaf with mixed raw veggies in a collard leaf wrap.
    - Salad with assorted raw and/or lightly steamed vegetables, nuts, seeds, and a simple olive oil and lemon juice dressing on the side.
    - Steamed assorted veggies (i.e. broccoli, cauliflower, green beans, asparagus, etc.) with chickpea hummus, almond hummus, or any homemade dressing you enjoy.
    - Sprouted grain wraps filled with mixed greens and legumes of your choice.
- **MORNING RITUAL** - Make it a habit of waking up half an hour earlier each day to prepare your teas, fresh juices, and smoothies. If you have all ingredients prepared the night before, you can even reduce this time to 15-20 minutes.
- **WATER** - Invest in a lightweight stainless steel or glass water bottle and get in the habit of taking it with you everywhere you go.
- **SUPPLEMENTS** - Purchase a small storage box for supplements from your local pharmacy and fill it up with all your needs for the week. Keep it with you at all times.

Building a healthy work environment requires more than just focusing on access to healthy foods. It's also about the physical surroundings and emotional aspect of life as well. When it comes to the physical aspect, apply the same tips and strategies as presented in the "setting up your home" section above. Make your workplace a clean, uncluttered, and inviting space whether you have an office or just a small working area. Setting up a Himalayan salt lamp on your work desk can help relax you and freshen the air. Having a bottle of peppermint essential oil handy is another great tool to invigorate you when needed or to get rid of a headache. Simply place 3-4 drops on the insides of your wrists, rub them together, and then use your wrists to massage your temples while avoiding contact with your eyes. Relax your body and breathe in the scent of the oil. It works like a charm!

The most crucial aspect, though, is the emotional side of the workplace. Time and time again I see people completely miserable because of the place or the kind of job they are in. And I get it, as I have done so myself for many years. It wasn't until I put my love for myself above all else that I was finally able to let go of the paralyzing belief that money and job security were the most important thing in life.

I am not saying that they are not, but when they supersede your well-being, and you find yourself compromising your health and your future, it is time to do something about it and look for a better way.

Take a moment and go through the following questions below to help you get some clarity in this area of your life. Then decide if there is anything you may wish to change in a way that will better support you and your health goals.

- Are you excited to go to work or are Monday mornings the most dreadful time of the week for you?
- Are the values of your co-workers and the company's aligned with yours?
- Do you feel like you are growing or do you feel stuck and not able to utilize your full potential?
- Are you constantly challenged to grow and do more, be more?
- Do you feel supported and encouraged or undermined most of the time?
- Do you see yourself working there in the next 5 to 10 years?

In my corporate job, I used to work an average of 80 hours a week, and I couldn't wait for Saturday night to come so I could finally have a day to do what I loved. I couldn't wait for the next vacation so that I could escape from my responsibilities. I now work 100 hours a week and can't wait for the next day to come.

When you build a life you love, work will no longer feel like a chore, like something you have to do. That is when you stop counting the hours, and you stop looking for a way to escape. You only have one life, so live it the way you want to. In the words of the late Wayne Dyer, make all your dreams a present fact by building a life that you don't need a vacation from.

Chapter 5.3

SABOTAGE IS INEVITABLE

Trust and have faith in knowing that what is meant to happen will happen at the time that it is meant to. Just keep working. Keep trying.
Keep putting forth your effort.
Make mistakes so you can learn from them.
Allow yourself to really enjoy the process of growth and learning and don't spend too much time wallowing over your little setbacks along the way.

—JENNIFER WARDOWSKI

One of the first principles I shared with you in this book was the idea that the most important thing to focus on is your journey. It is imperative that you slow down and learn to enjoy every step on your path. Whether good or bad, every experience is meant to teach you something that will bring you closer to your goals.

The reason it is so important to focus on enjoying and trusting the journey and the process is that doing so will help you get past any unexpected roadblocks. I can guarantee you with utmost certainty that at some point in time, in one way or another, you will mess up somehow and sabotage your success. Again, this is not a matter of "if" but "when." So it is best to prepare for it right now and not wait to react in the moment.

Every client I ever worked with, every person I ever interviewed, every role model I ever followed and I included, we all messed up at one point or another. It is inevitable. It is a natural part of the process and nothing to be worried about. Before we dig deeper into figuring out how to deal with this, let's look at a few examples of how sabotage can appear so you can recognize it and deal with it quickly:

- You may skip your daily exercise, finding an excuse that something else is more important.
- You may find yourself being distracted by a challenge that one of your friends or your partner, family member, or child is going through.
- You may skip your green juice or smoothie in the morning and then tend to overeat later in the day.
- You may tell yourself you do not have time to do the things you love.
- You give into your cravings and eat something that doesn't serve you.

The good news is this: because we know this is bound to happen, we can do something about it now before it happens. Plan and don't react. Decide right now that when sabotage shows up, you will be ready; you will know what to do. The key is to prepare ahead of time by developing an arsenal of strategies to be able to pull yourself out of a funk and back on track to achieving your health goals. There are three particular types of occurrences that can push someone off track:

1. Distractions
2. Sabotaging thoughts
3. The meaning given to intense emotional events

Let's look at them one by one and learn some ways to identify them and stop them in their tracks.

1. BEWARE OF DISTRACTIONS

Distractions destroy action. If it's not moving you towards your purpose, leave it alone.

—JERMAINE RILEY

One of the most common phenomena I observed over the years is the "slow motion" effect that distractions seem to have on us. These are sources of sabotage that we must be most wary of as they creep from nowhere, slowly but surely, like a snake hunting for prey. One moment you see them, the next you don't. It is because they are not something big that you see coming from a mile away. Rather, they are small actions piled on top of another like a snowball effect. They start small, and before you know it, their effects have trickled in throughout all areas of your life.

So what are your distractions? They are things you do to keep yourselves busy, things that you make more important than they really are. Here are a few examples to give you some clarity. A distraction can be:

- A long to-do list that you never seem to be able to get to the bottom of.
- An uncontrollable need to answer every phone call and check every email or to say yes every time someone is asking for help with something.
- A friend who constantly invites you to places not aligned with your new virtues and goals.
- Watching TV or spending too much time on social media.
- Giving too much focus to chores around the house or mundane tasks in your day-to-day life.
- Organizing your closet one too many times.

This is not to say that to-do lists are bad or that we shouldn't do our daily chores. Rather it is about living with purpose and living consciously rather than living in reaction to people's needs and events around us. We must remain at all times focused on our goals and adjust our paths as often as necessary to get there.

Whatever your potential distractions may be, begin by becoming aware of them ahead of time so when the moment strikes, you are ready and prepared to kick them out of your path as quickly as possible. Remind yourself as to why you are doing this and what it means to you. Thank your body and your mind for supporting you and remember that every new moment is a new opportunity to grow. You have the power to let go of anything that does not serve you.

2. BEWARE OF SELF-SABOTAGING THOUGHTS

Stand guard of the door to your mind.

—JIM ROHN

Self-sabotaging thoughts are similar to distractions in that they tend to show up unnoticed. You find yourself zoned out into an endless array of seemingly innocent thoughts that all together can form powerful limiting stories about what you can or cannot do. Days go by, and before you know it, you give into a craving, you forget to pack your lunch, you have one too many drinks, or you eat one too many cookies.

One of the best ways to approach this is to constantly be aware of what you are planting into your mind and your imagination. Be more proactive and become an observer of your thoughts and feelings. They are not you; they are a construct of your mind and thus they can be changed.

Make time every day to consciously focus on creating more positive thoughts with as much passion and enthusiasm as you feed your body with the best of nutrition. In Chapter 6 we will take a deeper dive in this area and I will share with you some of the best tools I have learnt for getting out of a funk and back on track.

3. BEWARE OF INTENSE EVENTS AND SITUATIONS AND THE MEANING YOU GIVE THEM

The kinds of events I am referring to here are completely different from your day-to-day distractions. These are the random "once in a while" type events that can come out of nowhere like a powerful wave. These are unexpected events like losing a job or going through a break-up or a severe illness. Be very wary of the meaning you give to such events and remember that there is always a lesson in whatever may come your way. Powerful life lessons always hide behind such events and it is your mission to find them, to understand them, and to use them for becoming a better and stronger person.

Under such circumstances, it is best to allow whatever time you need to process and heal and return to your path whenever you are ready.

Remember, your path is never lost and you do not have to start from scratch. That is not possible because you have already left hundreds of crumbs behind you through the actions and strategies that you have implemented already. Those are not lost. You also know in which direction you are heading due to the beautiful work you did in getting clear on your goals and the reasons for taking action towards their attainment. You can pick up from where you left off any time you choose.

KEY PRINCIPLES FOR STAYING ON COURSE

Here are some core principles for staying steady on your course and not letting distractions, thoughts, or external events slow you down or stop you.

- **Let go of perfectionism**
    - Who decides what perfect is anyways? It is better to fall a hundred times rather than not to do anything at all.
- **Keep adapting**
    - If you fall, get up as often as you need to. If a strategy no longer works, change it. If the second fails as well, change it again. Never stop until you get something that works for you and helps you grow.
- **Have faith**
    - Believe in yourself and know that when you are truly committed to something, mysterious forces in the universe conspire to bring you the results you desire.
- **Let go of too many rules**
    - Rules are everywhere. Listen to many of those, and you may find yourself spending more time figuring out what to do instead of doing it. Allow yourself to mess up and break some rules every once in a while.
- **Build a foundation**
    - Take a step-by-step approach to build a strong foundation for future success. A strong base of health will be there to support you and help you reach any goal you desire.
- **There is no such thing as failure**

- You may not get the results you desire on your first few tries. This is the time to remember that there is no such thing as failure unless you create it. There are only results: great ones, poor ones, mediocre ones, etc. Your results at one point in time do not define who you are and what you are capable of. They are not permanent in any way. Learn whatever you can from them, then leave them in the past and move on to trying something else.
- **Avoid hovering at one step for too long**
  - If you see something is taking too long to learn, implement, or adapt to, then just move on. Let it go and come back to it later. Don't spend too much time on it as you are in danger of getting stuck. Set a time limit rule for yourself depending on what works for you and follow it to the letter. Keep trying different things until you find what you enjoy the most.

Whether you get off track for a day, a week, or a few months, a strong health foundation will always be there, waiting for you. So when the time comes, and you find yourself off course, don't panic. Just breathe, relax, and start looking for clues to find your way back. I promise you that if you've implemented the strategies shared already in this book, you will find your way back in no time.

On your journey towards reaching your optimum health zone, remember to always *enjoy the process* and not focus on results that are less than what you desire. Move away from feeling like a victim and focus on what you can learn. Grow in knowledge and wisdom from every experience of sabotage, and you will transform that experience. The best part of reaching any goal is not the goal itself; it is the journey you went through to get there and the person you grew to be in the process. That's where all the great moments, memories, and magic truly come from.

STEP 5 – Key Takeaways

1. Choose the very first thing you will do on your journey to your optimum health. Will it be adding a daily green juice, getting a rebounder, or cleaning up your kitchen of processed foods? It doesn't matter what it is or how small. All it matters is the act of doing something to set you in the right direction. Small actions taken consistently are much more powerful in the long term than big actions taken only a few times.
2. Whatever it is that you choose to do, remember to not focus on results and the fact that you may not know how this will all work out. Just focus on celebrating that you have stepped up your game and are making progress.
3. Begin to notice all the things or people in your environment that are making it harder for you to follow through (e.g. not having a juicer, a non-supportive family member, lack of access to healthy foods at work, etc.) Once you know what these challenges are, you can begin to tackle them one by one. You must no longer accept anything in your life that is stopping you or slowing you down from reaching your optimum health zone.
4. In the process of trying new foods (i.e. raw juices, smoothies, etc.) you may begin to feel some changes and maybe even feel a little worse, to begin with. No need to worry; just know that your body is changing and needs some time to adjust to a higher influx of nutrients. Thank your body for having supported you for so long and promise that moving forward you will never let it get back to that state again.
5. Set yourself up for success by building a supportive environment at home, with your peers, at work, and where you live. Make it known to everyone that things are about to change and ask for their support.
6. Get to know all the places in your city where you can access healthy foods and wellness services: restaurants, juice bars, health stores, farmers markets, health clubs, yoga studios, detox centers, etc.
7. Surround yourself with people that have mastered their health and model their mindset and habits.

8. Personal sabotage is a normal stage in the process of change. Don't worry about it; just be aware of it, forgive, and remember that every moment is a new opportunity.

STEP 6

BUILD A SUSTAINABLE LIFESTYLE

Chapter 6.1

DON'T GET OVERWHELMED YOU DON'T HAVE TO DO IT ALL

I am only one, but I am one. I cannot do everything, but I can do something. I will not let what I cannot do interfere with what I can do.

—EDWARD EVERETT HALE

The health and wellness industry often works to make the topic of nutrition incredibly complex. In reality, once you get past the jargon, it's relatively simple. You will be surprised that, with just a bit of understanding, you will be able to start enjoying the process and truly get the health and energy you desire and deserve. The trick is not to overwhelm yourself with too much information before you've had a chance to apply it and get used to it.

You may often hear the concept that in order to get results fast you must think big. While that may be the case in other areas of your life, in this case, it is best to think small. By this, I do not mean that you need to stop dreaming big or slowing yourself down from progressing. Instead, it is much easier and less overwhelming to do small things consistently and thus, accomplish big things long-term.

It's all about taking a step-by-step approach and accomplishing your goals in small chunks, one at a time. Don't think about tomorrow; think about now. Do not focus on whether you will be able to quit smoking or quit coffee tomorrow; instead, focus on making a small positive change right now, today. Focus only on your next first step and nothing beyond; one-step, one moment at a time. Before you know it, you will accomplish great things.

One of the wonderful people I had the pleasure of interviewing for the writing of this book was a close friend, Vedran Šaćiragić who came up with a fantastic concept called "The 100 Hour Journey to Get Fit." It's a brilliant program where you commit to 100 hours of fitness over a period of time. You can do ten minutes, half an hour, or an hour a day, depending on how much time you have and what fitness level you start with. What I loved about it was the idea of "block" time. It was 100 hours, not months, nor years. It somehow made it more manageable and doable. I did not feel like I had to kill myself in one day. Instead, I took it step-by-step; I did as much as I could, and I was ok with it.

When I asked him about the strategy he used to get himself to take that very first step, Vedran's answer was simple: "I asked myself the question: What can I most control right now to get results?"

The idea of looking for something you can control gives you a sense of empowerment and a push to get going. You can control your state, the amount of time you work out, the type of exercise you choose, etc. Remember, you are always in control, and you decide what your next step will be. If all you can do is ten minutes of walking, then that's all you do. Don't beat yourself up for doing less than what you think you should or less than what others do. Ten minutes is a whole lot better than doing nothing at all. It is best to do things that are aligned with whatever stage you may be at. It is far better to do a little bit every day than to overexert yourself in an intense one-hour program.

Here are a few key ideas to assist you in this process:

- Avoid shortcuts and take small steps, one at a time.
- Small actions taken consistently will give you exponential results.
    - For example, let's say that you have not exercised for a long time and are about to start a new routine. In this case, a 15-minute power walk done each day is much more powerful and will give you much better results than a one hour walk done once a week. Plus, when you look at your exercise routine this way, it is also much easier and enjoyable to do.
- If you want to take this concept and make it even more powerful, you can add a little bit more effort each day or week to your already existing routine. For example, in the case of the exercise

program, you can add one extra minute each day, or you can add an extra five minutes per day per week.
    - Example 1: Monday you walk 15 minutes, Tuesday 16, Wednesday 17, Thursday 18, Friday 19, Saturday 20, etc.
    - Example 2: Week 1 you walk 15 minutes each day, Week 2 you walk 20 minutes each day, etc.
- When you begin to learn new recipes and cooking techniques, buy only one cookbook and start with one recipe per week. Prepare it once or twice and avoid moving on to a second one until you are 100% comfortable with it. Once you have it under your belt, you can proceed to the next.

Whether it is an exercise program as in the examples listed above, or you are learning new recipes, trying a new health routine, or wanting to shift your beliefs, it all works the same way. Start with small chunks and add as you grow and get more comfortable. The key is continuous progress and a step-by-step approach. This is a sure way to get long and lasting results. Never compare yourself with others and always do what you know works best for you.

KEEP SWIMMING NO MATTER WHAT

The reason many of us feel stuck and are too afraid to make a change is that we base the possibility of our future experience on results from the past. The truth is that the past cannot dictate who and what you are going to be and do; only the present moment can.

Right now you can make a conscious decision that what you are capable of doing has nothing to do with what you did or didn't do before, nor with what your parents or friends or co-workers told you that you could or could not do. Remember the hospital story or the limiting beliefs of my family who thought I was too nice to be successful in business? Had I allowed the past and those limiting beliefs to serve as the basis for my decisions, I would not be in a position to be writing this book right now, nor would I have ever had the chance to reach my dreams of empowering people and helping them create healthy lives for themselves and others.

The most important thing at this stage is to stay focused on what you want and keep going no matter what anyone may be telling you. Some will test you to see how committed you truly are to your new decisions by challenging your knowledge. Others may unintentionally slow you down out of fear that you may get hurt.

I will never forget the moment I shared with my family my decision to switch to a vegan way of eating. I was told anything from the fact that my pre-existing anemia would get worse to even the possibility of dying. The phone calls and text messages full of worry and anxiety seemed to be never-ending. I stuck to my guns, and in less than three months I was able to prove them all wrong. After over twenty years of consuming red meat, animal organs, and hundreds of iron pills aimed at fixing my problem with anemia, I was finally able to take things into my own hands and show everyone what a human body is truly capable of if given what it needs.

My new clean and highly nutritious plant-based regimen allowed me to cleanse my body, build a healthy gut environment, and absorb the nutrients I needed. For almost my entire life my iron levels had been so low that I often ended up in a hospital for intravenous injections. After a short period of time focused on detoxifying and nourishing my body, my iron levels were within the normal range. And guess what? Shortly after, all phone calls and panicked text messages ceased and my family doctor, to this day, does not completely understand how all this was possible.

BREAKING THROUGH SOCIAL BARRIERS

Aside from family and friends, one of my biggest challenges came from the social and professional groups I was involved with. This is an area where many people have a really hard time sticking to their new routines. Social barriers can be some of the most resistant of all, but with some tweaks and tricks, you will see that there are ways to get around.

I will never forget the day when I arrived at work with a strange-looking jar in my hand filled with a liquid that resembled the face of the green cookie monster. At least, that's what my beautiful stepdaughter said as she was helping me prepare my drink in the morning. Looking back at that experience, I feel so proud of my ability at the time to pull through. My job was no ordinary workplace; I was the head of the food services division of one of the largest universities in Toronto. This was the 13th and last year of that career. Everyone there was used to drinking soft drinks, artificial juices, and some of the most acidic coffee in the world.

As I walked down the hallway towards my office, everyone stared at my drink in complete awe; some made funny faces and giggled among themselves and some quite surprisingly made it well know that they could never possibly drink such "green slime." The shock lasted for a few days, and it turned into quite a water cooler conversation. I was determined to stick to my guns and lead by example instead of crumbling under the pressure of the masses.

It was only a few months after, that I resigned from my job and moved on to a new career. What I remember most is not the number of people who laughed but the few who built their courage to come and ask me about the green drink just as I had done a couple of years prior with that magical raw bagel. I was planting seeds every chance I got until one day, not long before I left, one of the girls in the office showed up at work with her own green drink. It was a day I will never forget. The ripple effects were spreading and, in no time, the girls in the office were in a frenzy about sharing recipes for smoothies and deciding who was going to come up with the best flavor combination.

The magic of this story is that, years later, the seed I planted is still growing. Many of them went on to radically shift their lifestyles and head on the path to what I call optimum health. And it all started with the "green cookie monster" drink.

Whether you feel unsupported by the environment in your workplace, in social groups, or while eating out, here are a few tips and strategies that will help and support you along the way:

- Never go hungry to a party or event where you are most likely not going to have access to healthy foods; eat before or bring a snack.
- Inform your friends and family that you are making a change and let them know what you will be eating or not in the future. Let them know that you do not expect them to prepare for your needs but rather to respect them and support you the best they can.
- Always remember that whatever you are doing is for you and your future, not to please anyone else.

- If you want to influence someone, it is best to show him or her what to do instead of telling them what to do. So be a role model. Always do what you believe is right and let them see the results. You never know whose life you may change.

Chapter 6.2

YOU WILL FIND THE "HOW" WHEN YOU ARE READY

When the student is ready, the teacher will appear.

—VINCENT VAN GOGH

In order to build a sustainable lifestyle that will guarantee you long-term results, you must focus most of your energy on *what* you want instead of *how* you will accomplish it. If you cannot figure out how to do something, it is simply because you have not yet had a chance to acquire the necessary information. You don't yet have the necessary references to support you in finding a solution.

The biggest challenge we all face on our path to better health is when we allow ourselves to feel stuck or overwhelmed by not knowing how to resolve something or move on to the next level. We ask the *how* question over and over in our minds, and when no answer comes, we block ourselves and, as a result, we limit our ability to find an answer.

The key to making progress is to stay focused on *what* you want and to enjoy the process of searching for the solution. You see, something magical happens when you just go with the flow, when you stop trying to control things, and you just keep looking for new ways; you try this, you try that, and before you know it, you become more. You learn a new strategy, you try a new tool, and you don't give up when something doesn't work.

Whatever it is that happens on your journey, remember that these are the stepping-stones and lessons that are meant to help you become more. They accumulate, and they push you to become more until one day when you are ready. That is the day when all that you need to know to figure out the *how* will be given to you. The teacher cannot come when you are not yet ready to understand that which the teacher is meant to show you. The *how* cannot come to you until you have become the person that can put it into practice.

I remember a time when all the tools and strategies I needed to change my life and health had been there right in front of my eyes, but I could not see them. They were outside of my bubble, floating around unseen. I asked for help, but I did not receive it until I was ready. Small signals and flashlights of hope popped out here and there as if to lure me into finding them. It is clear to me now that, somehow, all the events of my life seemed to be orchestrated perfectly to help me get to where I am today. They were sprinkled around in perfect harmony, helping me find my way home.

These somewhat magical signs came from random sources. They came from people who said things to me that made me question my reality; they came from random magazine articles about healthy eating; they came from the university student that demanded more vegan and gluten-free options; they came from that colleague of mine who brought the raw bagel to work. The signs came from everywhere, slowly but surely guiding me to where I needed to go.

All of us are guided in the same way. Our job is to open our eyes and see the signs. Our job is to find someone who can point us towards the exit door, someone who can give us the key and show us the way.

Next time you find yourself in an "I don't know how" type of situation, try something different. Tell yourself that you are on your way to figuring it out and then open your eyes and look for the signs. Who or what is around you that can help? Is it a person, a book, a health store, a new restaurant, or maybe your customers, employees, or even your employer?

Stay focused on what it is you want, then tune in and open your eyes. The answers you need are all around, waiting for you to discover them.

Chapter 6.3

FEED YOUR MIND

The physician above all should keep in mind the welfare of the patient, his constantly changing state not only in the visible signs of his illness but also in his state of mind, which must necessarily be an important factor in the success of the treatment.

—ARTURO CASTIGLIONI

I once had a young lady come to me desperately asking me to help her improve her health. She felt weak, tired, and sad, most of the time and she didn't know what to do anymore. I reviewed her health history checklist, and nothing jumped out as being a major problem. She was young; she looked healthy, ate quite well, exercised, and she had been seeing other practitioners for a while in her attempt to get better. I wondered what it was that I could do to help her.

As she started describing her situation, it all became clear. This beautiful soul was making herself sick with a never-ending array of negative and limiting thoughts of self-doubt and unworthiness. The same negative thoughts every day and every night tossed around inside her mind had no place to go and nothing to do but grow bigger and stronger. She lived in a bubble of doubts and limitations, and she couldn't find her way out.

You see, when we live in a non-supportive environment, all that we experience is directly affected by what's inside that environment. It's the same thoughts, the same food, the same people, the same everything. How can you get a different result if you always use the same ingredients? You can't.

Imagine your body and the billions of cells that die every second as well as the new billions of brand-new cells that are born at the same time. The cycle never stops as more and more dead matter accumulates and is ready to be discarded. If the cleansing systems of your body are not working well, if they are not fully functional, then some of this dead matter will stay behind and eventually pollute the whole environment.[36] This is why a detox program is so important. It allows you to open the doors and do a good clean-sweep.

Our mind works in the same way. Instead of food and water we feed our mind something else. We feed it thoughts, all kinds of thoughts. We are not just what we eat and drink. We are much more than that. We are also the totality of the thoughts that we entertain every moment of every day.

Thoughts never stop; they keep coming and going like the thousands of cars on a highway. Sometimes there are new ones, but most of the time it's the same old ones that we toss around in our brain hoping for a different result.

Self-sabotaging thoughts tend to show up unnoticed and all together can form powerfully limiting stories about what you can or cannot do. Thoughts, beliefs, and stories will keep coming and coming like a waterfall. You can learn to stop them for a while through the practice of grounding or deep meditation, but in your day-to-day life, the only thing you can control is the choice as to which thought you will focus on. It is crucial to be on constant alert as to the kinds of thoughts that pass on the screen of our life at any moment in time and to consciously choose to focus only on the ones that serve you.

Remember, what you feed your mind is what you will become. Feed it poison and more poison there will be. Feed it love and empowering thoughts and you can change the course of your life.

There are a few ways in which you can approach this. Here are some key strategies that I found most useful and able to provide the fastest results:

- Make time every day to feed your mind positive thoughts with as much passion and enthusiasm as you feed your body with the best of nutrition.

- Read or listen to inspirational audiobooks, online webinars, or podcasts. You can do this when you are driving, taking the transit, cooking, doing laundry, etc.; the possibilities are endless.
- Subscribe to email newsletters in the areas of your interest.
- Watch documentaries about people who have achieved results similar to those you desire. See the Free Resources section of my web site (www.otiliakiss.com) for a list of some of the best documentaries in the area of health and personal development.
- Attend conferences, workshops, or join groups related to personal empowerment and heath.
- Practice meditation and grounding – there are thousands of guided meditation Apps and YouTube channels available at no cost.
- Have a few hobbies and do something you love every day.
- Keep a journal of gratitude and magic moments and take time at least twice a year to review.
- Stay away from negative people and negative environments and pay close attention to anything that you allow to enter your mind.

It is not only what you do every once in a while that matters. It is what you do consistently and relentlessly, never giving up even when it feels like there is no way out. When problems seem too overwhelming, change your focus from listening to your head and listen to your heart instead. This is the time to feed your mind positive thoughts, one after another as if nourishing and hydrating yourself after a long period of starvation. There is no "too much" of this. Flood yourself with love, good energy, and positive thoughts as much as you can, for as long as it takes, and your life will never be the same.

Recommended Reading: *Change Your Thoughts – Change Your Life* by Dr. Wayne W. Dyer

Chapter 6.4

BUILD YOUR RITUALS STEP-BY-STEP

Huge achievement is less about your genetics and more about your rituals.

–ROBIN SHARMA

One of the first new positive beliefs that I acquired on my journey to reclaiming my health was that if anything were a must for me, I would find a way to make it happen.

What does it mean for something to become a "must"? It means that you somehow become laser focused on what you want and you no longer allow any internal or external factors to distract you or hold you back from achieving it. I truly believe there isn't only one way to do this. There are many ways; the key for you is to know what you want and to choose the techniques that suit your unique lifestyle best.

One way to figure this out is by asking a simple question: "What would you do to achieve your health goal if, for whatever reason, you absolutely had to?" The idea is to pretend that it is a must and observe all the things, thoughts or daily activities you would need to change to be able to do the things you want to do. For example, let's pretend for a second that tomorrow you absolutely must take a half hour to do some form of exercise. You had never been able to do this before as you always thought you did not have time. In this case, you must pretend that you have no choice but to create that time for you. What would you do? What would you have to change? Here are some additional questions to help you out:

- Could you wake up half an hour earlier?

- Could you find a way to organize your work schedule better so that you can leave work sooner?
- Could you do this during your lunch break?
- If you are a stay-at-home mom, could you get creative and find a way to do this together with your child?

The truth is that the time is there somewhere. Switch your focus from finding the time to creating the time. We all have the same amount of time to play with. Some days we do more and some we do less. It is not because we have less time; it is because we used it differently. It is because we prioritized our tasks differently and because we decided that some things were musts and we did them.

Before you go on to the next section, take a few moments now and notice how you perceive time. Notice how you can begin to shift your thoughts and feelings about the things you'd like to accomplish by choosing to create the time for them instead of finding the time. Does it feel different? Can you begin to see how this simple shift in perspective gives you power over every decision you make? Time is a tool for all of us to use in a way that serves our goals and dreams. So make the time for what is important to you and for what lights you up and don't let procrastination, endless to-do lists, and other people's needs dictate the time choices you make.

THE "NO EXCUSE" METHOD

The biggest challenge I had on my path to better health was not drinking enough water. No matter what I did, I always seemed to either forget my bottle at home or drink something else because the water had run out. One day I got sick and tired of this and decided to take things to another level. The water bottle did not work. The sticky notes on my fridge, in my car, and on my computer did not work. And so I thought: "What strategy could I use so I that couldn't possibly avoid drinking water?" And then the answer came to me. A friend of mine had gifted me for Christmas a "Camelbak" backpack that I had never used, and that was keeping the closet a lot healthier than me. I decided to use it to put my "no excuse" method into practice.

I filled that thing up all the way to the top and carried it with me everywhere. I mean everywhere! I took it to work; I used it at home, in my car, at the movies. I was literally glued to this thing for several days, morning till night. My boyfriend laughed, my friends laughed, and I think even our budgies gave out an extra silly chirp when I walked by. And guess what? It worked! For the first time, I reached my goal of drinking two liters of water per day.

Now, don't worry; you won't have to do this for the rest of your life. You just have to implement a "no excuse" strategy long enough for you to build a new habit. For some, it may be as little as a few days and for some a little more. The key to success is to be aware that everything you do or don't do, everything you like or don't like, is a learned habit. You were not born that way; you learned it, and that means you have the power to change it.

BAD HABITS CAN BE REPLACED

I happened to have a meeting with a client today whose young daughter had recently been diagnosed with autism and was directed by a naturopath to switch to a new diet. She explained how she had been having a hard time feeding her, as the little girl did not take to the new flavors and textures. She wouldn't eat anything but muffins and pasta, in other words, simple processed sugars that research showed were directly linked to autism.

Her mother felt like she had no control over her food preferences and couldn't understand why her daughter wasn't keen on trying new things. One day I asked her: "If your child had been born in Alaska, what would she want for breakfast? Or if she had been born in one of the few remaining rainforest tribes, what would she ask for lunch?" She looked at me puzzled, not able to come up with an answer.

I had specifically used such extreme questions to help her understand one crucial thing. A child's background, his or her life in the womb, and the way they are raised for the first few years of their life have an enormous impact on what they perceive as normal, on what they like, crave, and are generally used to. This woman's daughter had been raised eating muffins for breakfast and pasta for lunch, and this is what "normal" felt for her. She had been trained to eat that way. A child born in Alaska might want fish fritters for breakfast, whereas a child born in a tribe might want a bug stew for lunch. But go and offer muffins to little children in the tribe and they are the least likely to enjoy them as their taste buds are not used to such sweet and artificial flavors.

The message to her was simple: that she could help her child by helping her re-learn new healthy habits. It was not too late, and it was not impossible, as she had thought. It would not be easy, but she could do it by being a role model herself and implement the changes as a family.

Take a moment now and think about your own life. Is there something you keep putting off? Is there something that you keep finding excuses not to do? If so, pretend for a second that you absolutely must do it. Pretend that you are cornered in with no escape and that you have to find a way no matter what.

What would you tell yourself to no longer give in to your excuses?

What would you do?

When you get your answer, commit to it, mark it on your calendar, and do it. This is the only life you've got, so make the best of it.

Chapter 6.5

ALWAYS HAVE A TRICK UP YOUR SLEEVE

There's no harm in hoping for the best as long as you're prepared for the worst.

—STEPHEN KING

After having spent over fifteen years in the corporate world, owning two businesses and balancing a busy career with my passion for learning and having a family, I learned a thing or two about getting more done in less time, balancing multiple projects, or finding the tools to achieve even greater results.

The one thing that can significantly increase your chances of success in accomplishing whatever health goal you may have is always to have a "Plan B." In order words, it is to create more than just one way to get something done. It's about being flexible in your approach and constantly looking for better and easier strategies. Here are some of the best tricks that I collected over the years either from my own experience or that of my clients. Give them a try and see what works for you or get creative and come up with your own.

STAY FOCUSED ON WHAT YOU WANT

Get in the habit of always focusing on what you *want to* do versus what you *have to* do. Overthinking about what you have to do creates unnecessary pressure that you do not need. Instead, by focusing on doing what you want, you will be able to put yourself first and take actions that are much more rewarding. Doesn't it sound much better to say that you *want* to exercise versus that you *have to*? Give this a try for a few days by writing the question "What do you want?" on a few sticky notes and place them in random places like your washroom mirror, the stirring wheel of your car, or on your computer. This simple action can be absolutely magical in helping you make better decisions for your life.

FIND AN ACCOUNTABILITY PARTNER

One of the best reasons for having a coach, mentor, or close friend to help you on your journey is to provide you with a different perspective on doing things. Sometimes we get too overwhelmed with details, endless to-do lists, and even perfectionism and it is so great to have someone on the outside to point out better and easier ways to get something done. Who do you have in your life that could help you out? Is it your partner, a friend or would you perhaps consider hiring someone?

BEAT THE CRAVINGS WITH AN ANTIDOTE

This is probably my favorite one of all as it allowed me to get over a lifetime addiction to coffee. The idea is that, if you have a meal or beverage that is too acidic, you can use an antidote to balance it out. In my case, there was a time in my life when I drank an average of five cups of coffee per day. Today I still enjoy it every once in a while, and I always make sure to take what I call an "antidote" after.

The antidote is meant to counteract the negative effects of coffee. In this case, the antidote is a double shot of wheatgrass, one of the most potent foods on earth. That is my rule; if I have a coffee, shortly after I must have the wheatgrass and drink lots of water. You can do the same by using fresh green juices and E3Live shots (highly nourishing green-blue algae liquid). In time, the more energizing and nourishing foods you enjoy, the fewer cravings for energy draining foods you will have.

DETACH AND LET GO

Develop a belief that every moment is an opportunity to do something better and learn to move on past any unsatisfactory results quickly. If you fall off the boat one day and indulge in a big slice of pizza, don't beat yourself up. Let go of any feelings of guilt, recommit to your goals, and do better next time. It is your next step that counts the most!

TAKE IT STEP-BY-STEP

Focus on one area or one new thing at a time to avoid overwhelm. Let's say you want to improve your hydration by drinking 2 liters of water a day as well as a few green juices and smoothies. The best way to get this done is to begin with one small change and repeat daily. For example, you can start by enjoying a 12oz glass of simple green juice (i.e. apple and cucumber) every morning. Do this for a few days before you add more juice or more ingredients. That will give you time to adjust to a new routine or new flavors.

Another way to apply this idea is in exercise (e.g. 10 minutes daily versus 1 hour weekly) and in creating an empowering environment at home. One week you can focus on improving the food choices available in your fridge, another on researching new recipes, another on changing your cosmetics line, and so on. Before you know it, you will be living a new and fabulous lifestyle.

USE THE "ON THE GO" STRATEGY

I always look for better ways to utilize my time and so when I discovered audiobooks I instantly fell in love with this new way of feeding my mind. My challenge of spending countless hours in traffic or transit had been resolved and turned into something I thoroughly enjoy. From utterly disliking every second of being stuck among hundreds of cars, I now cannot wait to be stuck in traffic so that I can enjoy my time alone with my books. They are my friends, my partners in crime; they are my source of inspiration and food for my mind. You can listen to audiobooks, webinars, and podcasts while driving, cooking, exercising, walking, doing laundry. There are no limits to what you can do.

BREAK THE RULES SOMETIMES

Living your life at the highest standard possible is one of the best gifts you can give yourself. Daily and weekly routines are fantastic ways to stay on track and get the results you desire. Never forget though to feed your inner child as well and to let yourself be a bit silly and have fun sometimes. Whether this means waking up in the middle of the night to drive outside the city and watch the stars or running around in the snow with your bare feet while indulging on frozen maple syrup lollipops (Yes, I have done that!), remember to always live your life to the fullest. Know in your heart that it is more than okay to go a little crazy sometimes. In the end, it is those magical moments that will stay with you forever.

REINVENT IT

As you go about learning new recipes and cooking techniques, using the "Reinvent It" technique from Chapter 4 works wonders in keeping you healthy while being able to enjoy the foods you love. Remember my IKEA cinnamon bun addiction? I knocked it off the radar with my fabulously redesigned spiced baked apples with coconut and vanilla cashew sauce. All it took was a bit of research and a few trials to create an even better experience. Remember: there is always a way if you are truly committed.

MAKE IT FUN & CELEBRATE

Last but not least, remember to enjoy every single thing you do and celebrate every accomplishment. Fulfillment does not come from just doing the work; it comes from taking the time to enjoy the fruits of your labor.

Remind yourself that everything you do is a gift to yourself. It is not an obligation; it is a choice. This is your life, and it can be everything you ever dreamed it to be.

Life is never the same when you can change fear for curiosity and challenges for fun discoveries. Everything that ever comes your way is there for a reason. It is there to teach you and guide you in the right direction. You are a vehicle to bring your life's purpose into existence. Spend your time in awareness, observing and being curious about everything around you. Expect happiness and happiness will come. Expect health and health will come. Look for the fun in every action and every action will become fun.

Chapter 6.6

YOUR EFFORTS ARE NEVER LOST

Strength does not come from winning. Your struggles develop your strengths. When you go through hardships and decide not to surrender, that is strength.

—MAHATMA GANDHI

The road to success is not always a smooth ride and not always a path of continuous progress. Sometimes we slow down, stumble or hit a plateau and thus achieve results we did not plan for. Has that ever happened to you and what did it mean? Did it mean that you failed or did it mean it was just a stepping-stone to learn from and move on?

Many of us give negative meanings to results we do not want by telling ourselves that we are not good enough or that we failed. If that ever happens to you, don't beat yourself up. We all do it sometimes, as personal sabotage is a normal stage in the process of changing and growing. The reason behind it is that we haven't quite stepped into our new shoes, our new lifestyle. We are just testing the waters, and when they feel too cold or too overwhelming, our brain subconsciously backs out.

The key to getting past this phase is to build routines and systems in your life that will support you and either hold you up or guide you back to your desired path. It's like building a safety net. You may stumble a bit, you may fall, but your net will catch you, and you'll be able to get back on the path in no time.

These safety nets are designed and shaped based on your unique circumstances. They will be there for you every time you need them to help you get out of a rut. The better you get at your new way of life, the less and less you need them until one day you do them automatically. It's like learning to drive a car. At first, it seems overwhelming as we attempt to focus on doing ten things at the same time consciously. And then one day we catch ourselves driving the car, sipping our coffee, singing along the radio tunes and having a conversation all at once. You don't even think of driving as your subconscious has taken over. The way to get to this magical place is repetition. Repeat your new habits as often as necessary to get the results you desire. This system is guaranteed to work, and the only difference between you and me may be just a matter of time.

When I start working with a new client, I know that at some point or another they will sabotage themselves to some degree. It is not a matter of "if" but "when." In a way, that takes the pressure away as I know it is coming and I can help them prepare for it. It's the moment when your brain goes: "Wait a minute! What is going on? This is not normal; this is not me!" This happens once or twice until you've done it enough times that it begins to feel normal.

The first step to getting over personal sabotage is to know that it is okay to experience it as a normal stage in the process of change. When that happens, bring your focus back to your goals and move on. Every second is a new opportunity, and the only thing that matters is your next step, not what you will do tomorrow or the week after or months and years later. The more steps you take, the more crumbles you will leave behind and the easier it will be to find your path again.

The worst thing to do is to allow yourself to feel that you somehow "wasted" or "lost" all the work you had done so far. The truth is that you can never waste what you have already done. You might slip a bit, but you can never return to the point where you started. It is not possible because, in the process of changing your lifestyle, you grew as a person, you changed, you acquired new skills, new knowledge, new beliefs, new habits, and even objects in your home like a juicer, a blender, and new cookbooks. All these things are still there, and they will serve as great reminders and support systems to help you get back on track.

STEP 6 – Key Takeaways

1. No matter where you are on your journey to better health, remember not to allow yourself to get overwhelmed. You do not have to know or do everything. Just take the very next step in front of you.
2. While in most areas of your life it is important to "think big," in the area of your health it is best to "think small." This means taking a step-by-step approach. Small actions taken consistently will give you exponential results in the long term.
3. At this stage, the most important thing is to keep trying new routines and to keep heading in the direction of your dreams no matter what anyone may be telling you. Just listen to your heart and keep going.
4. When you experience any challenge, stop focusing on *how* you will fix it; instead, focus on *what* you want the *outcome* to be. Focus on *who* you have to become. You will figure out how to resolve any challenge when you become the person you need to be to handle that.
5. Build healthy habits little by little:
    a. Use the "no excuse" approach to mess with your mind a little and show it that you are in control. If your mind tells you that you cannot do something, then, by all means, do whatever it takes to do that same thing. You are in control, not your mind.
    b. Always remember that habits are learned, and thus they can be unlearned. You are not a victim of your habits. Crowd out old habits by introducing new positive ones. Making changes in the area of your health is like learning to ride a bike. Once you get it, you never forget. So do not worry if one day you fall off the wagon; just get up and keep going forward.
6. Make time every day to *feed your mind* with positive thoughts even if it is just five minutes to start. Read or listen to personal development books, read your list of new empowering health-related beliefs, listen to podcasts, watch documentaries in the area

of health and wellness, etc. Audiobooks are amazing as you can listen to them anywhere you are, whether you are driving, cooking, cleaning, on your lunch, exercising, etc. The more you listen, the quicker you will begin to feel stronger and in control of your emotions.

7. Put yourself in *inspiring environments* as often as possible. Attend conferences, workshops, trade shows, or any other event related to personal growth and health mastery.
8. Take *time to relax* whether that is by meditating, going to yoga, walking in nature, or doing anything else that works for you. The key is to do a bit of that every single day, even if it is just a few minutes to start.
9. Keep a gratitude and magic moment *journal* so you can always remember all the amazing things that you have in your life. Make it a must once a year to review them and see your progress and the beautiful things you were blessed to experience.
10. Learn to *forgive* yourself quickly and let go of unsatisfactory past results.
11. Break *the rules* sometimes – let your inner child come out.
12. Make changing *fun* and *celebrate* every bit of progress no matter how small.

STEP 7

LIVE IT!
ENJOY IT!
SHARE IT!

Chapter 7.1

LIVE THROUGH INSPIRATION

When you are living the best version of yourself, you inspire others to live the best version of themselves.

−STEVE MARABOLI

Here we are in the final step of your journey. I honor all of you that have gotten this far as I know you are some of the few people out there who do what they say, who walk their talk. There is no force out there more powerful in bringing change to those around us than the invisible energy that radiates from people who live their purpose, who walk their talk, and who live their life on their own terms. Some call it charisma, some call it confidence, and some call it passion. What I believe is that at the root of all these and more is something else, something much more powerful. Charisma, confidence, and passion are the secondary symptoms of *a source of energy* that feeds them. It is this source of energy that feeds you and allows you to be and do anything that you set your mind to.

Any of us can tap into this invisible energy feed any time we wish, but it's not as simple as asking for it or demanding it or taking shortcuts. There are laws that govern its access, and in order to abide by such laws, you must become aware of them and understand their mechanics. You, my dear friend, through the words of this book, have received your own private access to everything you need to know for reaching this source. It is up to you now to apply all that you have learned and reap the benefits.

There is no question that you can tap into this resource. We are all born connected to our own source of energy. Unfortunately, many of us unwillingly break the cord by making the wrong choices, by feeding our minds, bodies, and souls with foods, thoughts, and behaviors that do not serve us.

The good news is that you can reverse this process and rebuild the connection. You can open the portal to your source of energy by changing your habits and beliefs and going back to your roots. You begin by eating organic, clean, and highly nutritious food not as a new diet fad but as a return to tradition. We have forgotten our roots and our way of being aligned with nature and the universe. To escape our bubble, we must first realign ourselves with the universal laws of nature.

The quality of food you choose is important, really important but it is not everything. Feeding your body is not enough. You also have to feed your mind and your soul to truly step up your game. Life at this level is different than anything you may have ever imagined. You feel unstoppable and ready to tackle anything that comes your way. Your fears subside, and inspiration and passion follow you everywhere. People start noticing something different about you, but they cannot quite put their finger on it. They often remark that maybe you lost weight, or that you are glowing and vibrating with energy, and that somehow you look younger. They are in awe of your change and can't wait to ask you what you had done.

The most beautiful aspect of this new level of existence is not just about you. It is also the people around you. At this level, you have the power to plant seeds and help spread your energy to all those around that are ready to receive. Use your newly discovered power to spread inspiration and hope of a better way to everyone around you. Be a role model of all that is possible. Live always as the best version of yourself so that others can see and be inspired.

You don't have to do anything other than be yourself. At this level of existence, your energy radiates automatically and captures the attention of those who are open and ready. You can change someone's life forever by just being your higher self. You may do so with your presence, a word, your daily morning green juice, or a strange-looking dehydrated raw bagel. Sometimes that is all that it takes to make a world of difference for someone in need.

If you know anyone who needs help, your child, your life partner, a parent or a friend, know that the best way you can help them is by being the best role model there is. You cannot influence someone by worrying or stressing yourself out or by telling him or her what to do. You can only do so by *showing* them what to do. If you want to help someone have more energy, you must first be the energy. You must do everything possible to reach your ideal health zone and let that radiate from every cell of your body. Let them see the change in you right there in front of their eyes.

Let them see you.

It all starts with you.

Remember, one will not change until they are ready to change. The best thing you can do is to live as your best self right there, in front of their eyes. Love them, support them, and do not judge them. When they are ready, they will know exactly what to do, because, without even realizing, you have been their teacher all along.

Chapter 7.2

LISTEN WHEN YOUR SOUL SPEAKS

To make the right choices in life, you have to get in touch with your soul. To do this, you need to experience solitude, which most people are afraid of because in the silence you hear the truth and know the solutions.

−DEEPAK CHOPRA

"Don't tell me what to do. Don't tell me what I should or should not do. Don't limit me with your own fears. You cannot decide for me. Don't tell me I am too young or too old, too naive or too nice."

This is what your soul cries for every day of your life as it wants to grow and expand. We all have an innate desire built within us to do more and be more. It is this relentless desire and hunger that, when activated, can take you to unimaginable heights of success in any area of your life that you apply it to. You can be anything that you desire to be and never let anyone or anything limit you in any way; not your parents, not your friends, not the experts, not society or culture, and not your own negative patterns of thought. You can change all of that if you choose to do so.

You and only you have the power and no one else. All you have to do is tune into your heart and your soul as they are constantly challenging you to expand your horizons. Pay attention to your instincts and the things that seem to demand your attention. Pay attention to the things that appear to call to you and the things that don't make sense. Never accept something for what it appears to be. There is always, always something beyond appearance, something beyond thought, something more that you can aspire to do and become. It is all outside of your bubble, and there are unlimited resources to help you get there. There are people, situations, and events that come to you to help with the exact thing you need at the exact time you are ready for it. Just pay attention, listen to the cues, and act upon them.

If you don't like something, stop complaining about it and change it. Doing the same thing over and over again is not going to get you any better results. Pay attention to anyone around you who pulls you down and move on to find those who love you and support you.

Listen to the inner movement of your thoughts and do whatever it takes to keep the road clean. Feed your mind with positive thoughts and beliefs every chance you've got and never stop. Don't just try it once or twice; do it all day long if that's what it takes. Never stop until you get that which you desire.

At the base of all that you do, all that you are and all that you work towards is the state of your health and well-being. What you give it is what you get in return. The stronger your health foundation, the stronger everything else will be. Remember that health is much more than the mere absence of disease. It is the presence of an invisible source of energy that feeds every single cell of your body. This energy feeds into every action you take, every relationship you have, every job you do, and everything you ever dream to achieve.

Chapter 7.3

THE JOURNEY TO YOUR DREAMS

Every great dream begins with the dreamer.
Always remember you have within you the strength, the patience, and the passion to reach for the stars to change the world.

—HARRIET TUBMAN

If anyone had told me a few years back that I would ever live the life I live today, I would have thought they were kidding. In my wildest dreams, I could not have begun to imagine that it was possible to feel this way, to have this kind of energy and mental clarity. You really have to experience this yourself to truly understand, as words simply do not do it justice.

Whenever I begin a program with a new client, I always feel like I am burning inside with excitement and joy to share with them all the amazing things that are about to come their way: the energy, the joy, and the satisfaction of having completed an incredible journey. I await with anticipation their first cleanse, the early morning messages telling me how they had been able to get a full night of restful sleep for the first time in years, or the phone calls full of excitement to let me know of their latest breakthrough. I await with great anticipation their last blood work before the completion of their program and the time we take to check off the goals they set six months prior. There is no better gift in life than to see someone surpass their limitations and break free, to see the aliveness in their eyes when they can accomplish a dream previously thought to be impossible. I live for that!

Going through a process like this is not something to be taken lightly. It takes commitment, and it takes courage to dream and to keep pushing forward no matter what obstacles may come your way. That feeling we have when we achieve our goals is the ultimate place where we all wish to be, and truly it doesn't get better than that. And so, as we are about to complete our journey together, I would like to remind you of one thing. As I said at the beginning of this book, what will make you happy long term is not the achievement of the goal itself but rather the experiences you enjoyed during your journey and the person you became along the way. Goals, achievements and rewards come and go but what will stay with you forever is the feeling of fulfillment, joy, and gratitude for all that you have and all that you are. In the end, that is what truly matters.

    I feel blessed and honored every day for all of you that have opened up to me and shared a moment or more of your lives, your stories, and your dreams. And I am even more blessed to be able to live my life planting seeds of health and well-being in the minds of those of you who are ready and willing to become the best that you can be.

    It is your turn now to make the unimaginable imaginable. It is your turn to take things to a whole you level. I have played my part and handed you the key, the same way that my dear friend, Laura Luis, once did for me. The ripple effect continues. Take this key and leap into the future.

    All your dreams, desires, and goals are waiting for you.

With much love and gratitude,

Otilia

THE 7 STEPS – YOUR ROADMAP TO THE HEALTH YOU DESERVE

All you need is the plan, the road map, and the courage to press on to your destination.

–EARL NIGHTINGALE

I congratulate all of you that made it this far in my book, and I am truly honored to be able to play a part in your journey. I created the following list to serve you as a quick summary of the book, a map that you can use to guide you and serve you as a guide for staying on track.

STEP 1: WAKE UP! THIS IS THE ONLY LIFE YOU'VE GOT!
1. Step back and look at your life as an external observer and notice the areas that are not congruent with the highest version of yourself. Is there anyone or anything pulling you back?
2. This step is all about creating awareness and noticing how every single area of your life is so deeply impacted by the state of your health, your energy, and your mind-body-soul synergy.
3. Start paying attention and get really clear as to what beliefs you hold in the area of your health and how they make you feel.

STEP 2: LET GO AND SEE THE POSSIBILITIES
1. Get really clear on your health goals and the reasons why you want to achieve them. Review these on a daily basis to keep you on track.
2. Make a list of what you feel afraid of and what you feel is holding you back. Begin by becoming aware and curious about all those limitations and learn as much as you can about them. Can you begin to see the invisible bubble that has been holding you back?

3. Pay attention to new thoughts, ideas, strategies and objects that begin to show up here and there. The more open you are to them, the more of these will show up to guide you in the direction of your goals.

STEP 3: BUILD A STRONG FOUNDATION
1. Get really clear on what optimum health is for you and what the most common health misconceptions are. Then begin to apply this new knowledge in everything you do, from the food choices you make to the thoughts you choose to entertain.

STEP 4: PLAY TO WIN – PICK THE STRATEGIES THAT WORK FOR YOU
1. Whatever health challenges you may be experiencing, remember to distinguish between symptoms and the real cause. When the root cause is identified and eliminated, all symptoms can disappear.
2. Focus on developing strong hydration rituals to include living and supercharged water and other nourishing liquids.
3. Remember that the key to unleashing your highest energy potential lies in the quality and quantity of nutrients you ingest. It's not about being vegan, vegetarian, following a gluten-free diet or counting calories. The secret lies in maximizing your nutrient intake from real nourishing foods.
4. Make meal choices that allow your body to maintain the ideal alkalinity.
5. Develop daily, weekly and annual detoxification routines to help your body's healing mechanism work at its best.
6. Find a type of exercise you enjoy and make it a part of your weekly routine.
7. Keep your negative stress levels in check by incorporating whatever tools you need to stay grounded.

STEP 5: PULL THE ANCHOR AND LEARN TO HANG ON
1. This is where you begin to lay the foundation of the changes you are about to make. Set yourself up for success by creating an environment that supports you whether at home, at work on in social gatherings.

2. Self-sabotage is a normal phase that we all go through. Welcome it as an integral part of your journey and learn from it instead of letting it slow you down.

STEP 6: BUILD A SUSTAINABLE LIFESTYLE
1. Take a step-by-step approach to avoid overwhelming yourself with too many new things.
2. Focus on what you want to do versus on how you will do it.
3. Focus on feeding your mind not just your body.
4. Develop daily health rituals to help you build a sustainable lifestyle that can withstand any challenge that may come your way.
5. Remember that even if you get off course for a while, you can always find your way back. Your efforts are never lost.

STEP 7: LIVE IT! ENJOY IT! SHARE IT!
1. Listen when your soul speaks, as only it knows what is best for you.
2. Inspire and help others by living as the best role model you can be.

SO NOW WHAT?

So now what? Where should you begin? What is the very first thing you should do?

If there is one thing I hope you remember from reading this book is to keep things simple and just do something, anything! Taking any action no matter how small is better than doing nothing at all. Taking a small step every day will give you momentum and motivation to keep going. So here are a few ideas for things you can do right away:

1. Make a written commitment to your family and friends that you are embarking on an amazing health journey and ask for their support. You can do this via a post on social media or by simply calling someone.

2. Visit the Free Resources Section at www.otiliakiss.com and choose one of the recommended health and wellness movies. Schedule a movie night in your calendar right away and make it a family adventure if possible.

3. Take a drive to the nearest health store and buy a large stainless steel or glass water bottle, a few lemons and an organic green powder mix (look for something that includes dark leafy vegetables, herbs, and algae). This is a great way to kick-start your morning hydration ritual. Mix the juice of half a lemon and one teaspoon of green mix in 1 liter of water and enjoy.

4. If you do not already own a juicer or blender, do some research online into different brands and make a commitment to buy one as soon as possible. A great juicer and blender are the two most essential pieces of equipment you could ever own so get the best ones you can. You deserve it!

5. Begin by reading the book again. Yes, you heard me right; this is not a mistake. Doing something one time is not enough to create significant change. To move from mere knowledge to genuine understanding takes time and practice. So immerse yourself in this new world and keep feeding your mind. Reread the book, and this time mark down all the tools and strategies that called your attention and make a list that you can post in your kitchen or save on your phone. I recommend reviewing the book, especially steps 4 and 5, every month for the first year until this new knowledge is ingrained in your brain and it becomes your new reality. Trust me; it will be all worth it!

6. Block time on your weekly calendar for when you will be completing the tasks and exercises revealed in the book and commit to trying something new every week.

7. Be sure to visit www.otiliakiss.com and check out all the free resources available to you and join our community of health enthusiasts at www.facebook.com/otiliakisscoaching to get more inspiration and support along the way.

As I said at the beginning of our journey together, this book is meant to inspire you and ignite in you the desire to stretch beyond your comfort zone and expand the realm of what is possible for you. It is my sincere wish that the words of this book have given you a glimpse into what is possible for your life when you make your health the biggest priority. I honor all of you that have gotten this far, and I wish you a life of health, wealth, happiness, and fulfillment.

To your best health,

Otilia Kiss

ABOUT THE AUTHOR

OTILIA KISS is a passionate Wellness Advocate, Public Speaker, Author, and Certified Integrative Nutrition Health Coach. When she suffered from poor health a few years ago, Otilia quickly adopted the mantra "food as medicine" and completely healed herself from the inside out. After working for Fortune 500 Companies in the food & beverages industry for nearly two decades, she decided to go back to school to learn everything she could about health. Today, Otilia is here to help others achieve optimum health through the art of healthy cooking and holistic nutrition.

Currently, Otilia is the Founder of her very own company called Otilia Kiss Coaching where, as the "No Limits" Coach, she inspires and guides people to master their mindset, emotions, and health. She also serves as the in-house Health Coach and Co-Founder of Thrive Organic Kitchen and Café, an all-organic vegetarian restaurant dedicated to the health-conscious individual. In addition, she serves as a member of the Board of Directors of the Toronto Power Group, a personal development group with the goal to inspire and empower people to live the life they truly deserve. As a Public Speaker, Otilia inspires individuals, groups, and organizations to take their leadership and results to the next level by helping them break through the limitations standing in the way of their greatest potential.

Furthermore, Otilia received her Integrative Nutrition Health Coach Certification from IIN (Institute for Integrative Nutrition), a Bachelor of Business Administration (BBA) from Trent University and is now in the process of obtaining her NLP Practitioner Certification. She has also studied the world's top experts on peak performance, holistic nutrition and mindset mastery such as Anthony Robbins, David Wolfe, Dr. Brian Clement, T. Harv Eker, Wayne Dyer and many others.

Both driven and equally as committed, Otilia Kiss is on a mission to empower people to awaken to their limitless potential and harness it for their greater good. Ultimately, she strives to provide lasting solutions to every client to help them pave the path to a happy, healthy life.

ACKNOWLEDGEMENTS

Looking back at my life's journey so far, my heart fills with gratitude and my soul is in awe as I notice the myriad of magic moments that happened along the way to shape me into the person I am today. Some of these magic moments came in the shape of beautiful souls that came to light my path and guide me to discover my true self and my purpose in this life.

This book that you are holding in your hands is the result of all the love, inspiration and support I received throughout the years from some extraordinary individuals. Words are simply not enough to describe my gratitude to everyone though I shall do my best to summarize those that made an unforgettable difference in the creation of this book.

To my parents, Mia and Vasile Kiss, thank you for challenging me to be strong and courageous. I couldn't be the person I am today without that. I love you both!

To my partner, David Perez, thank you for believing in me and for always being there for me. You are one of the most determined and patient people I know, and there is no one else I'd rather have by my side on my journey.

To my beautiful stepdaughter, Athena, thank you for all the love that you have shown me since we met, and for all the laughter and the magical adventures. You inspire me every day to keep going and spread my message of love and health to everyone around me. I love you to the moon and back a million, zillion, gazillion times!

To all my clients and those of you who shared some of your lives with me, thank you for trusting me and allowing me the privilege of being part of your journey. It is an honor to have met you all and thank you for allowing me to share your stories and help inspire those in need to take action and change their health and their lives.

To Dr. Ashima, thank you so much for guiding me on my healing journey and for believing and supporting me in my mission. It is an honor to have met you and I look forward to continuing to spread our love for holistic health for many years to come.

    Thank you to Anthony Robbins for bringing my true self out and showing me what I am truly capable of. But most importantly, thank you for the unbelievably magical and overwhelming love that you and your team had shown me on that rare occasion when I had the brief chance to meet you. Your love was the purest and most unconditional love I have ever known; it was a love that had the power to heal, and that is a priceless gift I am so honored to have received. Thank you from the bottom of my heart!

    And last, but not least, I would like to thank two very special friends, Laura Luis and Tammy Peix for being such an inspiration in my life. I have seen you in good times and in bad, and I was always in awe of your resilience and drive to get through anything. You literally are two of the most limitless people I know. Thank you for showing me the way to the life that I truly deserve.

RECOMMENDED READING

The list below is a recap of all the recommended readings listed throughout this book.

The Magic of Believing by Claude M. Bristol
As a Man Thinketh by James Allen
Wheat Belly by William Davis, M.D.
Your Body's Many Cries for Water by Dr. F. Batmanghelidj
The Blender Girl by Tess Masters
Optimum Nutrition for the Mind by Patrick Holford
The End of Diabetes by Joel Fuhrman
Superfoods by David Wolfe
The pH Miracle by Robert and Shelley Young
101 Natural Remedies by Laurel Vukovic and Natural Health Magazine
Change Your Thoughts – Change Your Life by Dr. Wayne W. Dyer

Additional resources to help you succeed are available at www.otiliakiss.com

Interested in having **OTILIA KISS** speak at your next event?

Contact us at:

www.otiliakiss.com

REFERENCES

[1] Mann, T., et al., "Medicare's Search for Effective Obesity Treatments: Diets Are Not the Answer." *American Psychologist, 62(3)*, April 2007, p. 220-233.

[2] Kris Gunnars, BSc., "6 Reasons Why a Calories is Not a Calorie," https://authoritynutrition.com/6-reasons-why-a-calorie-is-not-a-calorie/

[3] Joel Fuhrman, M.D., *The End of Diabetes* (New York: Harper Collins Books, 2013), p. 107-110.

[4] Patrick Holford, *Optimum Nutrition for the Mind* (London: Piatkus Books, 2007), p. 266-267.

[5] Joel Fuhrman, M.D., *The End of Diabetes* (New York: Harper Collins Books, 2013), p. 107-110.

[6] Robert O. Young, Ph.D., and Shelley Redford Young, *The pH Miracle* (New York: Hachette Book Group, 2002), p. 24-25.

[7] Joel Fuhrman, M.D., *The End of Diabetes* (New York: Harper Collins Books, 2013), p. 2-3.

[8] Brian Clement, Ph.D., NMD, LN, *Dairy Deception* (West Palm Beach: Hippocrates Health Institute, 2014), p. 181-188.

[9] "American Medical Association Tells Hospitals to Go Vegan Ban Meat and Dairy!" http://thatveganrecipe.com/high_protein_pages/american-medical-association-say-hospital-should-go-vegan.html?utm_source=FB-AMA-SHARE&utm_medium=FB_SHARE&utm_campaign=FB-AMA-SHARE

[10] Sandi Busch, "What Are the Dangers in Drinking Alkaline Water?" http://www.livestrong.com/article/370249-what-are-the-dangers-in-drinking-alkaline-water/

[11] David Wolfe, *Superfoods* (Berkeley: North Atlantic Books, 2009), p. 170-171.

[12] David Wolfe, *Superfoods* (Berkeley: North Atlantic Books, 2009), p. 2-4.

[13] Robert O. Young, Ph.D., and Shelley Redford Young, *The pH Miracle* (New York: Hachette Book Group, 2002), p. 142.

[14] Kris Carr, *Crazy Sexy Diet* (Guilford: Globe Pequot Press, 2011), p. 34.

[15] Heather Muñoz, "What Are the Dangers of Heating Cooking Oil?" http://www.livestrong.com/article/225217-what-are-the-dangers-of-heating-oil/

[16] Tess Masters, *The Blender Girl* (Berkeley: Ted Speed Press, 2014), p. 21-14.

[17] Markus Allen, "How to Read Codes on Produce," http://www.truthin7minutes.com/how-to-read-codes-on-produce.php

[18] Patrick Holford, *Optimum Nutrition for the Mind* (London: Piatkus Books, 2007), p. 29-42.

[19] Joshua Rosenthal, *Integrative Nutrition* (New York: Integrative Nutrition Publishing, 2007), p. 214-219.

[20] Brian Clement, Ph.D., NMD, LN, *Dairy Deception* (West Palm Beach: Hippocrates Health Institute, 2014), p. 41-46.

[21] Andrew Weil, M.D., *Eating Well for Optimum Health* (New York: Random House, 2000) p. 87-88.

[22] David Wolfe, *Superfoods* (Berkeley: North Atlantic Books, 2009), p. 229.

[23] David Wolfe, *Superfoods* (Berkeley: North Atlantic Books, 2009), p. 40.

[24] David Wolfe, *Superfoods* (Berkeley: North Atlantic Books, 2009), p. 40.

[25] Kris Carr, *Crazy Sexy Diet* (Guilford: Globe Pequot Press, 2011), p. 23-24.

[26] Kris Carr, *Crazy Sexy Diet* (Guilford: Globe Pequot Press, 2011), p. 2.

[27] Robert O. Young, Ph.D., and Shelley Redford Young, *The pH Miracle* (New York: Hachette Book Group, 2002), p. 14-15.

[28] Kirsten Hartvig, N.D., and Dr. Nic Rowley, *You Are What You Eat* (London: Judy Piatkus Books, 1996), p. 64-66.

[29] Michelle Schoffro Cook, DNM, DAc, CNC, *The Life Force Diet* (Mississauga: John Wiley & Sons Canada Ltd., 2009), p. 10-11.

[30] Rosamond Richardson, *Organic Home* (New York: DK Publishing, 2003), p. 114.

[31] Dr. Phil Maffetone, "The 180 Formula: Heart-rate Monitoring for Real Aerobic Training," https://philmaffetone.com/180-formula/

[32] Norman Cousins, *Anatomy of an Illness* (New York: W. W. Norton & Company, 1979), p. 65.

[33] Michael T. Murray, M.D., *Stress, Anxiety, and Insomnia* (Coquitlam: Mind Publishing Inc., 2012), p. 67-71.

[34] Richard M. Sharpe, "How Strong Is the Evidence of a Link Between Environmental Chemicals and Adverse Effects on Human Reproductive Health?" http://www.bmj.com/content/328/7437/447

[35] Gillian B., "These 10 Deadly Chemicals Are Found in Most Body Care Products!" https://www.davidwolfe.com/10-deadly-chemicals-found-body-care-products/

[36] Kris Carr, *Crazy Sexy Diet* (Guilford: Globe Pequot Press, 2011), p. 96-98.

Made in the USA
Middletown, DE
15 July 2017